SEX EDUCATION FOR GIRLS
A PARENT'S GUIDE

SEX
EDUCATION
FOR GIRLS
A Parent's
Guide

Practical Advice on Puberty, Sex, and Relationships

Vanessa Osage

ROCKRIDGE
PRESS

To la niña atrevida,
the sunrise, the wind, and the rain.
All my Love

Interior and Cover Designer: Carlos Esparza
Art Producer: Meg Baggott
Editor: Nora Spiegel
Production Editor: Ashley Polikoff
Production Manager: Martin Worthington

Author photo courtesy of Heather Alvis

Paperback ISBN: 978-1-638-07710-7
eBook ISBN: 978-1-638-07544-8

R0

CONTENTS

PART IV
FREQUENTLY ASKED QUESTIONS, ANSWERED 127

INTRODUCTION

It's a fantastic time to be raising a girl.

As you'll see in the coming chapters, embracing this season of parenting can have positive impacts on girls and the people who love them in so many ways. Yes, the world is complicated today. The internet and social media present a whole new set of issues many of us did not face as children, and we can only imagine what it's like to come of age during a global pandemic. It is not the same world we grew up in, yet we can still walk alongside our daughters with power and grace. In this book, we will explore the many challenges girls face—both new and enduring—as they reach sexual maturity today. This book will strengthen you with information on a wide range of topics related to girls and sexuality, from talking about menstruation and safer sex, to promoting healthy relationships and supporting our LGBTQ+ kids. It will fortify you with practical tips, exercises, evidence-based research, and plenty of encouragement for the road ahead. I hope it will bring you ease and confidence. While the task of raising a girl through healthy sexual maturity can sometimes feel overwhelming, rest assured: you are not alone.

In addition to being a fellow parent of a daughter, I am also a Certified Sexuality Educator (CSE) through Planned Parenthood, with over a decade of experience teaching comprehensive sexuality education to ages 6 and up. I've worked with all genders and orientations, guiding young people and their parents through some of the most tender and profound topics that shape a lifetime. I've been a consultant; a birth doula; a professional coach in love, sexuality, and human connections; and a featured speaker at events, gatherings, and universities around the Pacific Northwest. For ten years I was founder and executive director of a nonprofit for puberty rites of passage, bringing support and celebration to sexual maturity in America.

First, I offer you what I ask of every participant in my classes, talks, or seminars: *respect.*

I understand that, whoever you are, you arrive to this moment through an entirely unique life path. I am grateful you are here, taking action to offer your daughter, perhaps, something greater than what you had in your own sexual development.

For some of you, the earlier chapters may be a review. Or you may find the information familiar, yet with a fresh take that helps you see things in a new way. I invite you to hop around and go where you feel most drawn. While the content is specifically tailored to parents of prepubescent and teenage girls, I trust you will find relevance here even if you are getting a head start and seeking information for a much younger girl.

Whether you have birthed your child, adopted your daughter, or promised to raise her as your own through marriage/partnership or another relationship, I want you to know that I hold this journey with the same reverence I do any major life transition. I understand that sexual health will look many different ways, depending on who you are and your family's goals and values. No matter who you are, I hope you will find what you need here.

The World Health Organization (WHO) defines sexual health as "a state of physical, emotional, mental and social well-being in relation to sexuality; it is not merely the absence of disease, dysfunction or infirmity. Sexual health requires a positive and respectful approach to sexuality and sexual relationships, as well as the possibility of having pleasurable and safe sexual experiences, free of coercion, discrimination and violence." We will use this as a starting point and courageously explore what all this means in the life of a girl.

I am excited to offer this retrospective of the most useful lessons I have distilled in over a decade of professional sexual health education. Regardless of your child's assigned sex at birth, their sexual orientation, your family structure, your religious beliefs, or any of the myriad ways we identify as human beings, *welcome.*

I am so glad you are here.

HOW TO TALK TO YOUR DAUGHTER ABOUT SEX

Let's just start by saying this is new and scary ground for many of us. In my work with parents, I've found that the majority would agree with this statement: "I did not have helpful information about sex and relationships when I came of age."

Many of us entered this realm through a cloud of secrecy and misinformation. Of course, today kids face the flipside of that challenge: easy access to too much information, only a small percentage of which is accurate or useful. We need to do our best to establish early on that we—not the internet, nor the whispered gossip of friends—are our child's trusted source for information.

As we dive in, let's keep in mind what I hear more than anything from adults in my sexual health work: "I wish I'd had this when I was a kid." Remember, you are giving your daughter this very gift.

The Challenge of Talking to Your Daughter about Sex

Why are these conversations so difficult? First, we're doing something very few of us had modeled: talking openly and honestly about sex. It can be hard to trust a practice we haven't seen in action. Fears of encouraging early sexual behavior and navigating our own social conditioning are just the beginning. Add the unknowns of supporting girls with varying abilities, gender identities, and sexual orientations, or those whose image is often exploited in the media . . . it all equates to understandable concerns.

Luckily, research illustrates why meeting this challenge matters. A 2009 international report by Advocates for Youth compares long-term outcomes in adolescent health by criteria of teen pregnancies, STD infections, and contraception use at first intercourse. The study finds that teens in France, Germany, and the Netherlands, where students often begin learning about sex starting in kindergarten, experienced better health outcomes than American teens in every category. Two things create greater, easier access to sexual health information and services for all people, including teens: 1) societal openness and comfort in dealing with sexuality, including teen sexuality; and 2) pragmatic governmental policies around sex education and birth control access.

The good news is that societal openness about sexuality can begin at home. Consider your family a micro-unit of society, where culture is created one conversation at a time. I invite you to see this moment as an opportunity to claim your own definition of what healthy sexuality can mean for your child.

The Importance of Sex-Positive Talks

As I mentioned, today's girls are growing up in an environment where access to information (and/or exposure to imagery) is more prevalent than ever before. According to research, the average age of first exposure to online pornography in the United States is now seven, and six worldwide. Additional research suggests that 88 percent of those images are categorized as "aggressive"—either emotionally or physically violent.

We need to talk to our girls in particular because they need a loving reality check about what sex is, and reassurance that their rights to respect, safety, and pleasure are equally important as anyone else's. One of the biggest surprises of this book may be just how early we do need to start talking—and parents are the ones who need to start the conversations.

Now, I'm going to ask you to do something that may seem entirely awkward in concept: schedule it.

Life is busy, and tricky conversations can be even harder to make time for once all the necessary business is tended. I recommend putting one topic per month on your calendar for the next 6 to 10 months. Then, find a time to discuss the topic sometime that month. You'll be glad you did.

You may get eye rolls or silence or even a slammed door (depending on your child's age). But fortunately, research confirms that our teens do hear us—we just need to be brave enough to talk and to listen.

Initiating Conversations

If we're lucky, we may get one or two direct questions from our kids about sex when they are very young. Otherwise, we have to set the standard for being the one they talk to. Try these points for easing into conversations:

It's okay to admit that you're nervous. Communication is 90 percent nonverbal, so it's best to acknowledge what they might be sensing as you begin. This also models healthy emotional intimacy. This might sound like, "I'm a little nervous to talk to you about this, but I care about you so much that I wanted to just start the conversation and do my best . . ."

Let her choose the time and place. This gives a sense of control and creates the best possible outcomes. "Hey, I'd like to talk about some meaningful things by the end of the week. What would be a good time for you? Do you want to get food after school and walk to the park?"

Consider responding to media as an entry point. While sharing a movie or television show with your daughter, the storyline can provide the conversation starter. "Wow, I noticed how forceful they were in approaching her. What do you think about that?"

Ask for her opinion in general terms. Young people often feel more comfortable talking about others first, before opening up about their true feelings. For example, you might try, "What are the kids at school saying about dating before high school?" Then, follow up with, "What do you think about that?"

Keep in mind that sharing highly personal details with a child can create a lack of safety. There is no hard-and-fast rule on what is appropriate. Just remember, these disclosures should help them feel less alone, but not burden them with information they can't handle.

Redirect very personal questions by responding to the deeper curiosity beneath the question. For instance, "How old were you when you first had sex?" can be addressed without revealing personal experience. "Are you wondering what is normal for when kids have sex?" Oftentimes, they need a reference point more than the specifics of your personal history.

Give her multiple safe ways to ask questions or seek support without the pressure or awkwardness of asking face-to-face. Let her know she can leave you a paper note in a special, designated spot, text or email questions, or even send an audio message. Then, follow up in person. Even when a bond is strong, sometimes a highly introverted child will need another way to connect. Temperament can play a role in choosing the best approach. Create a system of notifications that works for both of you.

Use a book to supplement (but not replace!) important conversations. Parents can introduce a great age-appropriate, sex-positive book and ask to have a follow-up conversation afterward. See Resources for a few great suggestions.

Be willing to do most of the talking, but allow space for your daughter to approach you. Don't expect a pubescent or adolescent girl to lead the conversation. These topics can feel intimidating, so remember that we are the ones setting the tone for a safe space to learn.

Allow awkward silence along the way. It's from this space that a girl might come forward with a doubt or concern she's been struggling with.

Fielding Questions

If you are fortunate enough to have your daughter approach you with concerns or questions, you've been given a great gift. Here are some basic guidelines, along with my "Three V's" (Voice, Vision, and Values) compass in talking to kids about sex.

Start with "Thanks for asking." This allows you to settle into the moment and reinforces an important fact: They chose to come to you for guidance. It demonstrates respect and encourages them to approach you again.

Find your Voice. Remember that communication is 90 percent body language and tone, so it helps to find your preferred voice in advance. Some people may imagine a warm and supportive grandparent or beloved teacher and mimic their tone. Choose in advance what you want to convey in your voice and stance.

Speak through your Values. Knowing your values around sex (we'll talk more about this in later chapters) helps steer the direction of your response. You can mirror back your daughter's values in your response to situations—for example, "It upset you when Sienna put Alicia down because you value respect," and "What do you think would be the more compassionate way to handle that?"

Hold your Vision of your daughter as you hope she will be later in life. This tool helps us keep our own systems calm and conveys a message of trust in her strength to grow into a remarkable, healthy young adult. Imagine your child as an adult of about 25, having sailed through adolescence with confidence, awareness, and self-respect. This keeps your response pointed toward the "true north" of where you are steering her as a parent.

Express your rejection of a behavior through your ideals and hopes. Conveying our values can be done on a spectrum from shaming to encouraging. Our girls learn a lot by how we speak of others. Be conscious of how you speak casually of others, so the door is open for her to discover her own identity and come to you for guidance again.

When expressing your values, speak about yourself primarily. As a continuation of this point, consider "That's heartbreaking for me, when people post that kind of language," versus "Those people suck." Your daughter may grow to fear your judgments of her if you speak harshly of others. Talking about ourselves is always safer.

If you don't know an answer, look for information together. This both reinforces that it's okay to not know something and also gives you an opportunity to introduce your daughter to reputable sites online for answering these questions.

HOW THIS BOOK CAN HELP

Sexuality encompasses a wide range of topics, and you may feel unsure about where to begin. It may be helpful to go right to the topic you feel most nervous about and start creating comfort by familiarizing yourself with it now. We all have places where an issue feels more "alive" or raw, so let this book be a way to integrate some of that energy into powerful conversations with your child.

If you want to know that you are not alone right away, you might enjoy browsing the Frequently Asked Questions, Answered section at the end of the book (page 127). You'll find references to chapters with more information sprinkled throughout.

Even if you believe your daughter is past a certain phase, be sure to revisit topics such as consent, boundaries, and encouraging girls to express wants, needs, and desires—as these are skills that benefit us at all stages of life.

Inversely, even if your daughter is very young— congratulations on planning ahead!—you will benefit from starting with what feels relevant and looking toward the time when you'll be grateful you are ready. Remember, "early and often" is the mantra when it comes to talking to our kids about sex.

If you're looking for simple language to guide you into conversations, feel free to browse the "Open a Dialogue" sections in chapters 4–17.

PART I

WHEN GIRLS GROW UP

One goal of this book is to offer you a holistic, well-rounded overview of what happens for girls as they become women. The process, of course, is highly unique—depending on your child's gender expression, assigned sex at birth, cultural and religious background, family structure, and more. The important reminder here is that sexual maturity and puberty entail far more than simply physical changes. They are a time of identity formation, social/emotional changes, and discovery of the world beyond the family.

Context determines so much of what we learn. I've always wondered about students in classes where sex education is relegated to a highly nervous and reluctant science or physical education teacher. If we teach sexuality in an isolated and nerve-racking environment, what is the message?

Alternately, if we fold these physical changes into an integrated view of who we are, what might we gain?

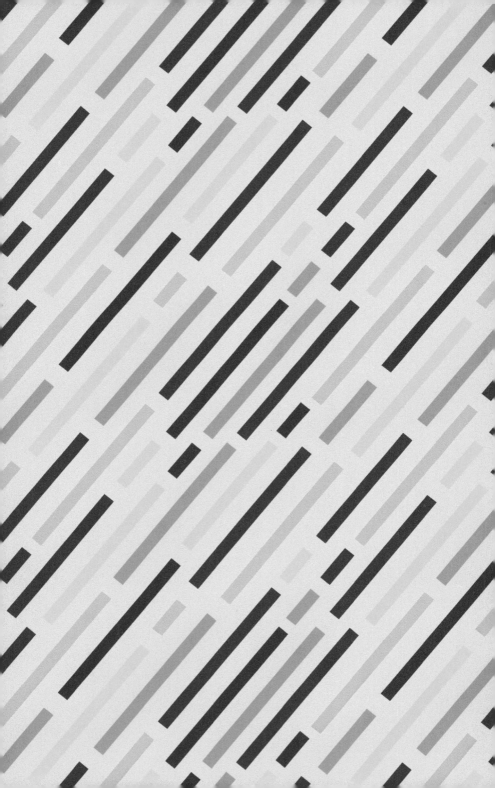

CHAPTER ONE

A Primer on Puberty

We'll start by discussing the physical changes
that typically happen during puberty for children
assigned female at birth. Generally, this means
development of the secondary sex characteristics,
such as breasts, labia, uterus, and ovaries. We'll also
begin to explore their development as it relates to
gender and sexuality.

    If your child experiences gender dysphoria and
is undergoing puberty blocker treatments, or if your
child is intersex (born with genital or reproductive
anatomy that does not fit in the binary of male/
female; about 1 in 500 births), developmental time-
lines will naturally differ.

    Wherever you are and whatever experience lies
ahead for your child, I hope this chapter will be highly
informative.

Going Through Puberty

Anytime we talk about the changes of puberty, it's important to remember that there is a very wide range of *normal*. Kids will often worry most about whether their body is "normal." It's a primary concern that can last for years. Labia majora (the outer, fleshy skin folds of the sexual anatomy for most people assigned female), labia minora (the inner, more textured layers), breasts, nipples, areolas (the darkened skin around a nipple), and body hair all come in a wide range of natural variations. Be prepared to reassure your daughter that her body is healthy and normal many times along the way.

Of course, some variations may warrant medical attention, and any true concerns need to be brought to your family doctor. Just keep in mind that your daughter may need gentle, ongoing reassurance.

Not only do physical expressions of the body vary widely, but the timing of these changes unfolds on a broad spectrum of normal, too.

Puberty can begin anytime from ages 8 to 14 in most kids assigned female. The process itself is a long arc of gradual changes that take many years to come to fruition. Your daughter may notice pubic hair first or have a growth spurt. Breast buds could be the first sign, or it may be widening of the hips. In the first stages, changes are happening internally, with the ovaries growing larger in response to the influx of estrogen in the body.

Generally speaking, girls are starting puberty (including menarche, the first menstrual period) earlier than they were decades ago. For example, in 1995 in the United States, the median age of menarche was 12.1 years old. Between 2013 and 2017, that dropped to 11.9 years old. Statistically, it may not seem like a great difference. But, looking back shows us the trend over time: Menarche occurred at age 16 or 17 a century ago—and today it occurs at age 11 or 12. You'll likely notice stories among other parents of seeing the signs much earlier than they expected.

Changing Sizes

A growth spurt often happens for girls 6 months to a year before their menstrual cycle begins. According to researchers at Johns Hopkins, growth in height happens at a rate of about 2.4 inches/6 cm a year throughout childhood. Growth slows slightly at the start of puberty, then spikes to about 3.14 inches/8 cm a year during puberty. If you pay special attention to your child's height, this may let you know changes have begun.

Many kids will experience "growing pains," an aching usually in the legs, shins, back of knees and/or front of thighs during puberty. These tend to be worse in the afternoon/evening (sometimes causing distress overnight) and ease by morning. Growing pains do subside naturally as the body reaches new levels of growth.

Adequate rest and nutrition are the best approaches, as the requirements during puberty are higher than at other times in childhood. You may notice your daughter's appetite increase, sometimes with strong cravings for certain foods for weeks at a time. As long as she is healthy for her size, you can trust the instinct to support the massive growth that is happening.

Changing Shapes

In addition to height, girls will gain weight and notice a new shape in the thighs and hips. If a girl is self-conscious about her weight or sensitive to social pressures to be thin, she may need reminders that the body is wise enough to reserve stores for her to grow into. You can reassure her that a growth spurt is underway, and her body needs nourishment to reach her full shape as a woman.

Some of the changes may be welcome, and some may feel scary or overwhelming to your daughter. A lot depends on her timing and what she sees happening in the girls around her. Girls who develop earlier can feel fear of a process that is happening beyond their control, while those who develop later may experience frustration or embarrassment at feeling "left behind."

Puberty is often a time when transgender children experience increased stress, panic, and possible gender dysphoria (a sense that their bodily changes do not align with their own gender identity). They will need special care, acceptance, and support to navigate this time well (see chapter 17 [page 120] and the Resources section [page 138] for more information).

Puberty is an ideal time to model self-acceptance for our girls. It may seem like your affirmations and messages are falling on deaf ears—but they do hear you. For some parents, witnessing our children's sexual maturity will resurface old, unresolved feelings about our bodies as we grew. Consider it a chance to see this natural process through newly matured and loving eyes. Offer your child a greater level of acceptance of her body than you may have had available for your own.

It's okay to validate how uncomfortable the changes can be. Admitting that you (may have) struggled too takes some of the edge off the isolation a teen can feel. Just be sure to conclude your reminiscence with lots of reassurance, offering the perspective of time. We can use words like "healthy," "normal," and "natural" to witness the process with acceptance together.

Hair

For some girls, the development of pubic hair can mark the onset of puberty. Darker, thicker hair will appear on and near the labia majora (the outer, visible folds of skin between the legs) anytime between age 8 and 13. It may appear first as one long, thick hair—or the natural hair of the skin will thicken gradually from the center. Hair also appears under the arms and may thicken on the forearms, thighs, buttocks, and back as well. It is one undeniable, visible marker of the changes to come.

Keep in mind, Americans have a funny hang-up about pubic hair. Girls may face pressure to be smooth and hairless as their bodies mature. You may want to talk to your daughter about hair removal—and make sure she understands the choices available to her. Hair removal practices tend to be passed on from women to girls, and parents of all genders have the opportunity to encourage their puberty-age girls to do what feels comfortable for them, whether that is shaving or letting their hair be.

Skin

The influx of sex hormones that inspires the new growth of hair can also lead to acne and other skin problems in teens. The skin is the largest organ of elimination, and nearly every teen will experience changes in their skin as their bodies adjust to these fluctuations. Many skin conditions can be treated primarily by healthy hygiene habits and staying thoroughly hydrated. Clean, healthy foods and adequate water support the process of elimination, healing, and recovery for so many systems in the body.

Be aware that a whole industry exists to respond to a child's anxieties about acne and breakouts. While these moments can challenge a child's sense of security from time to time, products with toxic chemicals to treat acne can actually cause further problems in the long term. Please see the Environmental Working Group's database of products to understand their impacts on the body (see Resources, page 138). Raw honey is a wonderful alternative for treating many topical skin conditions, with many of the same antiseptic and antibacterial properties as pharmaceutical products.

Overall, your daughter may need to be reassured that there is nothing wrong with her and that her body will regulate any skin issues over time. Talk to your doctor if you have concerns.

Breasts

Development of breasts is often the most outwardly noticeable sign of puberty's progression. For this reason, it can be the greatest source of self-consciousness or embarrassment for girls. A fitted undershirt or training bra can help minimize potential embarrassment. Breast buds—a small nodule of new tissue under the nipple—can appear anytime between age 8 and 14. Some girls will worry about the breast bud being a sign of cancer or other disease, so let her know in advance that this is completely normal.

Breast buds can be tender or sensitive, and the areola (the soft, pigmented skin surrounding the nipple) also grows in size and darkens at this time. The breast bud will develop first, followed by breast tissue—new nerves, blood vessels, and adipose tissue—in concentric growth over time.

One breast often grows more quickly than the other and generally balances out on its own. Breasts grow for at least four years, so a girl's shape at full maturity is not determined by what is happening along the way. As parents, we can affirm the inherent loveliness of all body types. Media preferences on body shapes may change over time, but the ideal body type is the one your daughter can love.

Body Odor and Hygiene

At puberty, the adrenal glands begin to secrete Luteinizing Hormone (LH) and Follicle-Stimulating Hormone (FSH) in bursts. In addition to inspiring the growth of underarm and pubic hair, these higher levels will bring about body odor and oiliness of the skin. For a girl at puberty, nightly showers with natural soap will help regulate these effects.

If your daughter wants to use deodorant, help her choose a product with minimal toxic chemicals; this is especially important when and if she chooses to shave underarm hair. The open pores at hair follicles can become an entryway into the body, so a non-toxic option is best.

The vulva and opening to the vagina are naturally self-cleaning and need no additional care beyond simple washing with natural soap—and only on the outside of the body. Your daughter may need to hear from you that douching is unnecessary and can actually disrupt the pH balance of the body. Her body is functioning naturally, just the way it is.

Vaginal Changes

The surge of hormones during puberty inspires the labia minora (the inner skin folds) to swell and enlarge, often "blooming" beyond the labia majora (outer skin folds). Girls may notice these changes and need reassurance that they are normal.

A surprising number of people have come of age without knowing that vaginal discharge, a fluid released from the vagina, is a normal and healthy part of their body. Vaginal discharge differs from the lubricating fluids that are secreted when the body is sexually aroused. At puberty, the body produces a much higher amount of estrogen, signaling the mucous membranes to secrete fluid to simply moisten and protect the vagina.

Most girls release about a teaspoon (4 ml) of vaginal discharge per day, and this amount can increase up to 30 times just before ovulation. Mucous becomes thicker and more slippery at midcycle, and a bit drier and tacky to the touch before menstruation. These are part of the signals we can learn to understand menstrual cycles.

About six months to a year before the first period, the body will begin producing vaginal discharge to prepare for menstruation. Glands lining the cervix and vagina create fluid that is clear, milky, or slightly yellow in color—fluctuating from thick to thin consistency with the phase of a girl's cycle. This will often show up inside the underwear and is entirely healthy.

Only if the color or smell changes dramatically is it cause for concern. Clumps of thicker white mucus could indicate a yeast infection, so it helps to teach a girl these symptoms. Overall, natural cotton, breathable underwear is best to avoid the risk of bacterial infection.

Menstruation

Menstrual cycles tend to start earlier for girls today than they did in the past, between age 11 and 15 for most girls. The average age of first period in her biological family (on both sides) can offer a clue on timing. Menarche, the first menstrual period, usually arrives about two years after breast buds appear.

Once a girl begins cycling, she may have anxiety about knowing when her period will start next. I encourage parents to consider teaching their daughters to track their menstrual cycles through temperature and charting. Basal body temperature is low at menstruation and rises near ovulation. This practice encourages self-awareness, supporting emotional and physical health. She will naturally learn to value her body in the process, while the record-keeping is useful for her medical health history (see Resources for suggestions, page 138).

Periods are usually irregular when they begin (for many months after menarche), and the fluid can appear as brownish or red. Girls need to know in advance that this can start at any time. Help her create a period bag of basic supplies (cloth and/or disposable pads, a change of underwear) that can fit inside a basic pencil case. She can keep this with her in the years when she awaits her first cycle. We'll talk more about menstruation in chapter 8 (page 71).

Understanding Gender Identity and Expression

We will explore this topic more in chapters 3 and 17 (pages 30 and 120), but for now, let's review the basics of gender identity and expression as they relate to puberty. *Gender identity* does not necessarily correlate with our sex assigned at birth (meaning our external genitals and reproductive systems) or who we like sexually. When someone's perception of their gender matches their sex assignment at birth, they are referred to as cisgender. When their perception of their own gender does not match their sex assignment at birth, they are called transgender.

Gender expression is not the same as gender identity; it's about how we present ourselves to the world. It's a choice we make about how to be on the outside. Someone may identify as female (cisgender), be attracted to males (heterosexual), and have a gender expression that falls more on the "male" side of social expectation. These expressions exist within a cultural context and are part of a young person's developing identity.

Many transgender people, though not all, become aware in early childhood that their gender identity does not match the sex they were assigned at birth. But puberty is when this awareness—and the unease and confusion that accompany it—becomes acute. For kids who experience an internal mismatch between their anatomy and their gender, the term *gender dysphoria* is used medically. The Mayo Clinic clarifies that gender dysphoria "might start in childhood and continue into adolescence and adulthood (early onset). Or, you might have periods in which you no longer experience gender dysphoria followed by a recurrence of gender dysphoria. You might also experience gender dysphoria around the time of puberty or much later in life (late onset)."

Again, please refer to chapters 3 and 17 (pages 30 and 120), and the Resources section (page 138), for more about gender identity and expression and how to support your child. Puberty can be a particularly tender time for transgender and gender-expansive children, so it is important for parents to be as informed as possible.

When Girls Develop Sexual Interest

In nearly every middle school classroom I've entered as a sexuality educator, I've seen a wide range of new interest in romantic or sexual relationships. A highly developed bisexual or heterosexual girl of 14 may already be boy-crazy and dating, while another girl of 13 may have zero interest. There is often a percentage of kids who focus more on fantasy worlds through literature and film to explore emotional depth, instead of engaging with a fellow classmate. Some will begin questioning their sexual orientation, while some may have held secret crushes for years or more.

Kids of preschool age (4 to 7 years old) are often first to show fascination with the anatomy of other people. A five-year-old will unselfconsciously blurt out at a party, "Does Uncle Jimmy have a penis too?" These questions aren't sexual in nature, but simple curiosity. Young children do experience sexual arousal physically and may discover masturbation on their own, as early as age five (or sooner).

Masturbation is a common, healthy activity. Plenty of research has confirmed the health benefits of the endorphins associated with orgasm, such as reduced stress, improved sleep—even relief from menstrual cramps, improved body image, and self-esteem. Masturbation allows young people to discover what they truly like and don't like—and is a foundation for very healthy sexual development (more about this in chapter 11 [page 86]).

As an aside, kids from ages 5 to 11 may also experiment with their friends as an expression of curiosity about bodies. Some generations may know this as "playing doctor." This can happen anytime between preschool and middle school—and is more common than most people realize. As a parent, discovering that your child has explored another child's body or shared their body with a friend can feel alarming initially. A whole host of fears may arise. This behavior happens among kids of the same or different genders and does not indicate sexual orientation or promiscuity.

The most important thing to consider is whether there were power dynamics at play—for instance, was one child older or in a coercive position? Feel free to calmly bring discussions of consent into this moment (see chapter 16 [page 114]). An age difference of even a year can contribute to discomfort in a child saying no. So, make sure everyone was in full agreement. If this arises in parenting, consider it an opportunity to lay a foundation for future sex-positive conversations while the stakes are still low. Curiosity about bodies is natural, so keep your language neutral, calm, and educational. Every encounter with the concept of sexuality can help your child frame sex in a positive way as they grow.

On a physical level, hormone levels will rise in all bodies at puberty, heralding an influx of estrogen, progesterone, and testosterone. With this, true sexual attractions may arise for the first time. These can be mixed with romantic or platonic longings. The best way to support our daughters is to take their romantic or sexual interests seriously, neither downplaying nor over-encouraging what they feel.

Remember how overwhelming new emotions are for toddlers as they experience them for the first time. Girls can be thrown off-center by the intensity of new longings—integrating each in their own time. A new world of physical sensations and emotions opens up to them at sexual maturity, and the path can be a beautiful one.

KEEP IN MIND

- We are the best source for truly supportive information about sex for our kids.
- Loving and accepting our bodies is a lifelong journey that requires special support and encouragement at puberty.
- Knowing they are "normal" is a primary concern for kids going through puberty.
- Parents need to be the ones to start conversations about sex.
- Supporting our kids to embrace a positive sexuality will usually mean stepping out of our comfort zone as parents.
- The courage to start honest conversations now will pay off in profound rewards for both parent and child in the years to come.

CHAPTER TWO

How Should a Woman "Be"?

Now, let's pan back to look at the wider cultural and social forces that can influence a girl's coming of age. We raise our girls now on the blessings of earlier waves of progress—from women's suffrage in 1919, to civil rights protections in the 1960s, to financial freedoms for women in the 1970s—but many of the same pressures and expectations remain. This includes new ones exacerbated by the internet and social media. When it comes to raising a healthy, confident young woman today, the crucial factor is whether or not she accepts the messages she sees about female sexuality.

Mixed Messages and Double Standards

Sexual maturity is the time when girls begin to internalize messages about what it means to be a woman. Social acceptance beyond the home is a primary developmental task, and they are looking for clues. These tend to come primarily from media, group affiliations (such as church, sports, or other social networks), and friendships. Your daughter is likely highly aware of power dynamics now: Who makes the decisions? Is a girl celebrated or condemned when she complains of mistreatment or injustice? Who manages the money and why? Whose career takes precedence in the family?

So much of what girls see today causes confusion about their role in relationships—or distances them from the truth they experience in their bodies. We can help them come back home to their true selves. I often tell parents in my seminars and discussions that sex is everywhere in America—but nowhere we need it to be. The void in the conversation is often filled in with unhelpful and even dangerous messages. As parents, we need to fill that void with messages that reinforce the health and value of mutual pleasure in sex.

Outside pressures can influence how a girl experiences closeness with a loved one, the vitality of her body, and soon, the dynamics of her chosen family. We'll take a look at each of these forces to guide us in facilitating higher levels of health for girls today.

Whether it is thinness, agreeableness (an inclination to not set boundaries), submissiveness, or extreme selflessness, girls today are likely managing a lot of external expectations to be a certain way—one that often separates her from herself. It's important to help our daughters recognize the microaggressions that are used to keep girls quiet and in line.

Remember, society may offer up a whole appetizer plate of unhelpful messages to our girls—but our daughters still get to decide whether to take a bite or to order more of what is being served.

Let's examine some of those messages more closely . . .

"Girls Are Responsible for What Boys Do Sexually"

It may have started with Eve in the Garden of Eden story, but modern Western society has a long history of blaming women for the behaviors of men. Interpersonal responsibility is a basic foundation for healthy human relationships. Knowing who is responsible for what creates clarity and a framework from which people can grow, regardless of their gender. To achieve clarity, we need to dissect the current confusion.

Rape Culture is a set of ideas that perpetuate social norming of sexual violence. It can include absurd and subtle notions such as a girl's clothing dictating a boy's behavior, blaming the harmed person instead of the one who acted abusively ("She asked for it"), and demonizing regular human activity when done by one gender instead of another. Society may rush in to discredit a woman when she speaks up about abuse. Some brush aside a boy's abusive or harassing actions and speech by saying things like "Boys will be boys," or "It's just locker-room talk." The function is to get certain men "off the hook" and place undue burden onto others—allowing the behavior to continue unchecked without accountability.

We can raise our daughters with the clear awareness that they deserve to be treated with dignity and respect (and for those with sons, to share this lesson as well).

"Sexually Active Men Are Players, but Sexually Active Women Are Sluts"

Back when women were considered legal property of their husbands, the idea of a woman even enjoying sex threatened to disrupt a patriarchal power structure. At one time, controlling sexual behavior was an underlying attempt to preserve a social and power structure in favor of male dominance. Unfortunately, remnants of this unhealthy paradigm still linger today.

If a man enjoys multiple sexual partners (consensually or not), he may believe it somehow confirms his manhood or earns him the societal nod of approval. If a woman enjoys many sexual partners, she might expect a decrease in positive social regard. Even those women who endured unwanted sexual advances from men were somehow burdened with stigma. The double standard is that sexual activity may increase a man's perceived value while the same (even unwanted) activity can potentially decrease a woman's.

Yet, the reality is that for healthy, empowered couples today, both partners enjoying their sexual experiences leads to the greatest overall satisfaction. When a woman does not or cannot enjoy sex because of fear of "slut-shaming" or double standards, everyone loses. Sex therapists are often the most overbooked professionals in the mental health industry. Clearly, we all need another way. Helping your daughter grow toward freedom and pleasure within her own values is a great contribution to societal well-being.

Whose Story Are We Seeing?

Here, we have a chance to trace mixed messages back to their source. To help your daughter critically examine the messages she receives about women, you can teach her about the Bechdel Test. Created by cartoonist and cultural critic Alison Bechdel, this shockingly simple three-point assessment determines whether a film has achieved representative gender balance:

1. The picture features at least two women (bonus points if they have names).

2. The women talk to each other.

3. They talk about something other than men.

It's laughable when laid out this way—yet a stunningly high percentage of films do not pass the test. Examining how many shows in the top three genres of 2021 (according to Netflix) pass the Bechdel Test:

Comedy (less than ½)
Animation (barely ⅓)
Drama (less than ½)

Notice that only a third of U.S. animated films popular with children pass the Bechdel Test. That is cultural conditioning in its earliest stages. This simple tool can help explain to girls of many ages why they may be seeing enactments of sex that do not embrace mutual pleasure or equality.

Talk to your daughter about whose story you are seeing. You can even check for the name of the director and/or producer and ponder together what we might see about love, sex, and relationships if it was "her story" and "our story."

THE SUBSERVIENCE OF FEMALE PLEASURE

Men have held disproportionate control of the media industry for decades, and the resulting "male-centric" storytelling lens has strongly influenced ideas about the value of male pleasure vs. female pleasure in sexual experiences. It also perpetuates confusion about what pleases a woman sexually (vigorous thrusting vs. clitoral stimulation; see Chapter 12 [page 92]), essentially leaving their preferences out of the conversation.

Healthy conversations about sex on-screen—even between heterosexual couples—are incredibly difficult to find. Our girls may only ever see media that prioritizes a man's pleasure over a woman's—along with all the imbalanced dynamics leading up to these sexual moments. The risk is, if she wants to be desirable to a man, a girl may conclude this is the role she must play. Given how private sex is, and how eager young people are for guidance, how can we give her alternate messages?

In addition to educating our daughters about their anatomy and sex, it's important to engage with media in a discerning way together. If you are watching a movie with unrealistic or harmful depictions about relationships or sex, ask your daughter questions like, "Do you think she really wanted that?" Include comments like, "It doesn't look like this is about her satisfaction, does it?" The critical lens will help equip her with media literacy skills and a new way to question what she sees.

The Emotional Life of Girls

Research shows that all genders experience the full range of human emotion—it's only cultural conditioning that limits their expression for certain gender identities. For girls, freedom to verbally or physically express emotion is greater in all but the emotions of anger and pride. These are more readily expressed by men. Again, it is not the *experience* of the emotion but the *expression* that varies by gender.

Girls also often receive a message that they are "too emotional," implying that the forces moving within them cannot be trusted. Worse, they run the risk of denying their emotional responses in decision-making—separating from their own deepest knowing.

We need to unteach this equation:

emotional = unreliable = less worthy of consideration

If we want our girls to trust themselves and navigate the world with confidence, we have to support their emotional self-acceptance and teach them to trust the wisdom of their bodies. A "red flag" about a situation or person is often first felt in the body. Consider reflecting with your daughter about her social encounters by asking questions like "How did your body feel in that moment?" or "What is your gut telling you?" It's an opportunity to help her cultivate a relationship with her body as an ally.

If our daughters can learn to embrace what they feel—from emotional reactions to gut sensations—they can eventually guide themselves toward the kind of sexual experiences that truly support them. In her book *The Four-Fold Way*, Angeles Arrien, PhD, observes that "in wilderness survival training, they always tell you, 'When in doubt, trust the body's intelligence, because the body will not lie.'" Applied to parenting for healthy sexuality, this framework will help our girls navigate their own lives for both safety and pleasure.

Mood Swings

Emotional intensity happens now for girls (and all genders) in a way that echoes that of the toddler years. They experience a similar sense of overwhelm, with an underlying question: *Will I always feel this way?* The rush of greater hormone levels, along with a broader understanding of the world and the self, creates moments of profound emotionality. This is normal and healthy, within reason.

When our daughters are in the throes of big emotions, two major elements contribute to her success in moving through. First is her ability to accept the new feeling as normal and healthy— knowing there is nothing wrong with her. Remind her that this new intensity is okay, that her body and heart (if you use that language) are expanding now. She will learn to regulate in time. Just normalizing big emotions can eliminate any added anxiety or thoughts of *What's wrong with me?*

Second is our ability to remain steady as parents. Our job is to hold a safe space—without becoming emotionally entangled. It is a supreme challenge of parenting teens (of all genders) to remain a calm, supportive witness to their experience. We offer reassurance without minimizing what she feels, and we support her agency by resisting the urge to swoop in and try to fix everything for her. Think of it like the winds that rock a sailboat in the storm. We hold the lines steady, keeping the passengers secure, and remind new sailors that storms do have a peak—then they pass. They roll through. We can weather this one, too.

Remember, demonstrations of a rageful "I hate you!" from behind a slammed door are not necessarily indicators of their respect for you as a parent (or a human being). More likely, it's an expression of the need for an anchor in that storm. They only need to know you will be there, regardless of what they are going through.

DEPRESSION AND ANXIETY

According to research published in *JAMA Psychiatry* in March 2020, anxiety, depression, and other internalizing problems are becoming more prevalent among adolescents. "Externalizing" behaviors such as acting out and violence were more common in boys, whereas girls tended to direct their pain internally. The study references data from 2017 revealing that 20 percent of adolescent girls aged 12 to 17 had experienced at least one major depressive episode in the prior year (compared to 8.7 percent of adult women).

The Centers for Disease Control and Prevention (CDC) lists these signs of depression to watch for in adolescents:

- Feeling sad, hopeless, or irritable a lot of the time
- Not wanting to do fun things she previously enjoyed
- Showing changes in eating patterns—eating a lot more or a lot less than usual
- Showing changes in sleep patterns—sleeping a lot more or a lot less than normal
- Showing changes in energy—being tired and sluggish or tense and restless a lot of the time
- Having a hard time paying attention
- Feeling worthless, useless, or guilty
- Showing self-injury and self-destructive behavior

In addition, girls who are struggling with anxiety may exhibit the following behaviors:

- Feeling nervous, restless, or tense
- A sense of impending danger, panic, or doom
- Increased heart rate or rapid breathing
- Feeling weak or tired
- Trouble concentrating

- Having trouble sleeping
- Experiencing gastrointestinal (GI) problems
- Having the urge to avoid things that trigger anxiety

If your daughter shows these signs, it's important to learn more—or arrange for professional help. Do not wait. I encourage you to take your daughter's mental health seriously, as it affects every aspect of a girl's life. Suicide is now the second-leading cause of death for teens and young adults in America.

Connecting with our tweens and teens can be tricky; they need space and independence more than ever. Connecting with them deeply can be even more challenging. Our daughters may not act sad or talk about their helplessness, so we have to dig deeper. Reaching this level of understanding takes time, and we have to create the space for it to surface. Consider setting aside a regular time each week (a certain evening or weekend morning) as a chance to learn what is really going on in your daughter's life.

Sleep, Nutrition, and Mental Health

The importance of sleep in the teen years cannot be overstated. A 2013 Australian study confirmed that sleep deprivation adversely affected the mental health of participants aged 15 to 17. There was a direct correlation between those who got less than seven hours of sleep at night and emotional states described as "depressed, confused, or angry."

Limiting late-night screen time can improve your daughter's chances of reaching restorative REM sleep. Consider insisting that screens not be allowed in the same place that she sleeps. The blue light from devices disrupts her natural rhythms, interrupting the body's ability to regulate growth hormones (GH), especially important for growing bodies, and also oxytocin, the "love and bonding hormone," which is important for stress management and resilience at any age.

Experts in sleep recommend keeping a distinction of the bed as only for sleeping so that our minds don't associate it with other activities and energy levels. As much as possible, keep a consistent bedtime. This also helps the body regulate and enjoy more consistent replenishment during deep sleep.

A girl's digestive health is also strongly linked to her psychological well-being. The gut has its own nervous system (enteric nervous system) where bacteria regulate the release of neurotransmitters like serotonin and gamma-aminobutyric acid (GABA), important for mood regulation. The communication between the gut and the brain travels along what is called "the gut-brain axis"—and researchers found that supporting the gut through probiotics in patients with Major Depressive Disorder (MDD) led to a decrease in depressive symptoms.

If you are concerned about her mental health, and unsure of the quality of her diet, talking to a nutritionist could be the most effective way to get positive results.

Impulsivity and Risk-Taking

The adolescent mind is perfectly primed to seek out novel experiences, while understanding of the resulting consequences remains low. It is important for parents to be proactive in talking to their tweens and teens about substance use in its various forms, starting as early as age 10 or 11. When a child knows their parents' stance on recreational drugs and alcohol, they are far less likely to take excessive risks.

As a sexuality educator, I was surprised at how often questions about drugs and alcohol naturally came up in discussions around sex. Teens often associate forbidden substances with entry points into the legitimacy of the adult world. Without solid information about each substance from a reliable source (not an older teen or the media), how it affects the body, and whether it is a safe thing to try, kids are at far greater risk for impulsivity with substance abuse.

Just as with talking about sex and relationships, studies show that parents speaking calmly about substances in a fact-based way with their kids produces the best long-term outcomes. When studied longitudinally, conversations about drugs and alcohol that were categorized as "open and neutral/nonjudgmental" led to kids taking little or appropriate risks later in adolescence.

The Social Life of Girls

When girls shift focus from family-as-center to peer-group-as-center sometime around the age of 10 to 13, it is a healthy, natural, and developmentally appropriate shift. That doesn't mean it is easy for us as parents. It just means it's necessary.

They need to know they can survive in the world without us. That often means that some days they push us away—even bristling at every annoying thing about us. Then, other days, they cuddle up and share like the child we've always known. When I led coming of age programs for a puberty rite of passage, parents nearly always talked about how dizzying it was not knowing which version of their child they were going to get on any given day.

Expect to become especially embarrassing to your daughter as she grows highly self-conscious of her new place among her peers. Nearly all children of puberty age momentarily believe that "everyone is looking at them"—a kind of fishbowl perception unique to early adolescence. If a parent being their usual self disrupts their child's fledgling sense of identity, it can cause real upset. Prepare to step back when her friends are around and to approach her with more awareness and gentleness when she is at home.

Part of the task of adolescence is incorporating sexuality into their newly forming identity, and our daughters will crave privacy. But, they also need a whole lot of guidance when they can hear it. Try to look for signs that they are open to talking amid the push-pull of dependence and independence. For older teens aged 13 to 16, the shifts can be even more dramatic. A colleague in family support services put it best: "They don't need us—until they desperately need us *right now!*"

A Growing Desire for Privacy

Adolescents are involved in a deep process of identity formation during the puberty years. They are developing a well of inner knowing, and often facing some of the darker realities of human existence. They feel the scope and weight of the world more fully than at any time yet in their childhood. Psychologists often call this "shadow work": facing the darkness in ourselves and in the larger world, an essential component of developing a healthy sense of self.

This "going inward" can mean more time spent alone, distancing from parents and caregivers. Adolescents especially spend time in contemplation of their changing bodies and lives. Not wanting a parent to see them naked any longer most often is—instead of an expression of inherent shame—a claiming of their bodies as their own.

Our job is to respect their newfound privacy and resist any urge to make fun of or poke at their newfound vulnerabilities. Try to remember the courage it takes to face a group of increasingly important peers while you don't know one day to the next whether you'll have a new emotional overwhelm or new physical dimension (welcome or unwelcome!) to take with you.

Friendships in Flux

Some friendships enhance our self-confidence, while others can challenge it. Sexual maturity is a time for girls to learn more about these realities in relationships. So we can help our daughters examine the ways different connections impact their sense of belonging and place. The goal is to help her know her value, regardless of current social connections.

From age 11 to 14 or so, the important thing to remember is that change is the constant. One month (or week!) a girl may feel secure and surrounded by wonderful friends. Next month, it's uncertainty and doubt. She is lonely and longing. Then, a new connection sparks and joy returns. It's common for friend pairings and groups to change at this age, and it can be confusing and sometimes heartbreaking. It is not uncommon for the first major "breakup" a girl experiences to be with a best friend. (We'll talk more about friendships in chapter 12 [page 92].)

A helpful framework is to remind her of the value of keeping many good friends, and to focus on self-discovery. We can offer, "Okay, Callie is preoccupied with Isla now. It's sad because you miss her and value your closeness. What have you learned about yourself that you can carry into your other friendships?" (This is a great time for that values conversation!) "What do you know you need to feel truly accepted and connected to someone?"

Some friendships offer more laughter and play. Is this a value or a need of hers? Some are based on deep sharing and trust building. Talk about what supports her best. Discuss what works in each friendship, or what is missing. This helps her venture forth to forge connections anew. Don't be surprised, also, if Callie is back the next week with renewed vigor for connecting. The most important message is "You and your self-awareness are inherently valuable amid all of this, regardless of who calls you tonight."

THE ROLE OF PEER PRESSURE

When bodies and lives are changing rapidly, young people tend to do a lot of comparing and judging themselves for perceived differences. Yet, comparing up or down always leads to unnecessary pain. At puberty, it's more about a need for belonging than assessing one's value. She may be insecure that "everybody" is developing breasts when she is not (or the flipside—she may have developed earlier than most of her peers). She may believe "everyone" is dating, while she is not yet interested. This is a great time to help her normalize different rates of growth emotionally, socially, and physically. You might offer:

"This is a process that is unfolding, and everyone's timing is right for them."

"It's natural to notice what is happening for others, but it doesn't mean any one way is better than another."

"Wow, I noticed how your friend chose what was right for her, even when everyone else was doing something she was uncomfortable with. Isn't that wonderful?"

KEEP IN MIND

- Striving to be the "ideal woman" will only lead to pain for girls—encourage them instead to become their "authentic self."
- Remind her that her pleasure, her experiences, and her self-worth are just as valuable as anyone else's.
- Sit down and challenge the media you see together—she needs to know how to critically assess what she sees in film and online.
- Normalize emotional intensity so she knows there is nothing wrong with her as her life changes dramatically.
- Take time to learn about your daughter's well-being each week—and seek help if you have any concerns for her mental health.
- Practice role-playing scenarios that encourage her to stand up to peer pressure by trying out different ways to say no.
- Affirm her character development first and pay attention to her sense of self-love.
- Help her find the constant in the changing social landscape—her own self-discovery.

CHAPTER THREE

Gender, Sex, and Sexual Health

Today more than ever, sex education is more than explaining the fundamentals of sex. It's really about preparing and supporting your daughter as she grows into herself. Sexual health and wellness are a big part of who she is, what she stands for, and how she sees and interacts with the world. In this chapter, we touch on these concepts of selfhood so you can help your daughter actively and joyfully claim her own experience of sex and sexual wellness.

Gender Identity and Expression

A great place to start is understanding the distinction between sex and gender. So first, let's clarify these terms, as well as some related vocabulary. You may use this background to refresh your own education and, more importantly, to affirm your daughter's identity and expression. Perhaps she's showing signs of questioning her own identity—trying out different looks with clothing, hair, and accessories. She is likely connecting with friends and peers who are exploring their own identity. The exploration is part of the successful passage through adolescence. Let's get clear on language so you can help her make positive decisions along the way.

Sex: When referencing identity, sex is a physical concept based on genitalia and other reproductive organs. Sex can also be classified based on chromosomes and hormone levels: generally male, female, or intersex.

Intersex: This is a category given to bodies that display some combination of male and female physical characteristics. About 1 in every 500 births is intersex.

Gender: In contrast to sex, gender is a construct in the mind, revealed by behavior, social and relationship roles, and how each of these are expressed. Gender includes an individual's perceptions of themselves, as well as society's interaction with that perception. Think of the two in this context: sex is mostly physical and/or anatomical, whereas gender is primarily psychological, emotional, and social.

Gender identity: This is best described as the way a person feels and experiences their own gender. The exploration of gender identity can begin before puberty. For many kids, it takes fuller shape throughout adolescence, and well into adulthood. Gender can be identified as male, female, non-binary, gender neutral, transgender, agender, pangender, and genderqueer—all, none, or a combination of these. Help your child understand that it's okay for them, or anyone, to not categorize their gender identity. Also explain that gender identity can exist anywhere on that spectrum throughout a lifetime.

Gender expression: This is what people present to the world regarding their gender identity. It is how they *do* their chosen gender. Gender expression is the sum total of choices we make, including but not limited to clothing; hairstyle; jewelry, makeup, and other accessories; physical mannerisms; and voice. Let your child know that however they choose to express their gender identity is up to them and that they need to respect others' choices as well.

Gender dysphoria: This is the discomfort or distress that occurs when people feel a mismatch between their assigned sex and their gender identity. For example, a child assigned male at birth who understands themselves authentically to be female. Having a certain identity but expressing another—a misalignment of the two—can also cause a disconnect that could enhance gender dysphoria.

Cisgender: This is a term for anyone whose gender identity is the same as their sex or gender assigned at birth, or whose anatomy and gender identity align. You may come across the shortened term "cis," meaning cisgender.

Transgender: This is a term for anyone whose gender identity does not match their sex or gender assigned at birth. A 2016 report by The Williams Institute at UCLA found that an estimated 1.4 million, or 0.6 percent, of adults in the United States identify as transgender. In reality, that number is likely much higher.

Nonbinary (including **gender expansive**): This is a term for anyone whose gender identity does not fit on either the male or female end of the binary (one or the other). It also includes people whose ideas of gender expand beyond social norms, or who identify as a mix of genders. Those who are **gender fluid** experience their gender as changing over time; they may feel more female some days and more male on others.

Pronouns

Pronoun usage is an important part of validating someone's gender identity and lived experience. The two most common personal pronouns are binary, "he" or "she," which doesn't match everyone's gender identity. The most common non-gendered pronouns at the time of this writing are "they" and "them," in place of "he/she" and "him/her." Other common nonbinary or gender-neutral pronouns include the neopronouns ze or xe (substitutes for "he/she," both pronounced "zee"), and zir or hir (for "him/her," rhyming with "here").

Embracing this use of language allows your child to know that they have options in their identity and expression. That freedom is inherently valuable. It also helps cultivate openness and acceptance of peers. When in doubt, one can ask, "What are your pronouns?" or use "they/them" until advised otherwise.

This is somewhat recent cultural progress, and sometimes it's hard to understand. A few clarifications to keep in mind: 1) Expressing a non-female gender does not equate to an attempt at trying to get attention. 2) Taking a nonbinary pronoun does not equate to going through a phase. What is real for us is real in the present moment. Teens evolve as they age (as we all do), which means gender expression might change over time . . . or it may not, and that is okay and simply needs to be accepted. But lastly: 3) Your full acceptance of "real for you" for your child in each moment is precisely what allows that human being to become their full, authentic, and best self, regardless of identity, expressions, and/or pronouns.

Developing Sexual Interest

Sexuality is our unique imprint of attractions, longings, bodily awareness, and sensual awareness within the romantic, emotional, and spiritual elements of who we truly are. It is multidimensional and ever-evolving. Puberty is a time of dramatic change, and reaching sexual maturity is not a onetime event. This is one moment in the long unfolding of sexuality's fullness throughout a lifetime.

The development of sexual interest is also unique to each person—it may arise initially from a platonic (nonsexual) attraction to a longtime friend and suddenly deepen to include other desires around middle or high school. Hormones and their rise play a role in the timing. It's also important to distinguish that desire is often present long before the decision to act on the desire ever plays out. Some girls may have a strong romantic experience, feeling a desire for union with close or distant people (think, the teenage heartthrob). This is valid in and of itself. If you find your daughter expressing strong romantic or sexual desires in either writing or drawing between the ages of 10 and 14, this is most likely the natural stirring of a longing to be fulfilled further down the road.

When it comes to sexual orientation and attraction, the terms that follow will help with clear communication. Remember that while people aren't always accurately defined by labels—and identity can change throughout life—language can help a teen give voice to their emerging self-awareness.

Lesbian and Gay: When a person is attracted to those of the same sex and/or gender. "Lesbian" usually refers to women who have romantic or sexual attraction to women. "Gay" usually refers to men who have romantic or sexual attraction to men but people of all genders can refer to themselves as gay. "Homosexual" is now an outdated, offensive term because of the association with anti-gay speech or rhetoric.

Bisexual: Generally speaking, this is when a person is attracted to both the same gender and other genders, though not necessarily equally or at the same time.

Queer: A person whose gender identity, gender expression, and/or sexual orientation falls outside of the societal norm for their assigned sex. This is also the term used by many people as a catch-all or umbrella term for the LGBTQ+ community, or as a substitute for gay/lesbian.

Asexual: A person who experiences little to no sexual attraction. Asexuality is different from deciding not to have sexual contact with anyone (abstinence or celibacy).

Pansexual: A person who is pansexual is someone who is attracted to persons of any gender. Many people who identify as pansexual say their attraction is usually focused on personality, rather than gender.

Sex and Sexual Health

A broad and diverse vocabulary empowers young people to have informed discussions about sex, and to engage in safe, pleasurable sex when it is right for them. Below are a few important and inclusive terms regarding sex and sexual health to inform your conversations.

Abstinence: This is when a person chooses to refrain from having sex of any kind, not just penile-vaginal sex. Abstinence can be for a specific amount of time or over a lifetime. This is the only behavior that is 100 percent effective at preventing pregnancy and STIs. As a choice, it still allows for physical affection and social closeness.

Virginity: Originally a religious concept meaning "woman unto herself," this term has been adopted casually to refer to someone who is yet to have (usually heterosexual) intercourse.

Oral sex: These are sex behaviors that include mouth to vulva, mouth to penis, or mouth to anus. Some young people may think that oral sex isn't technically "sex." That definition may vary from generation to generation, but one thing to keep in mind is that oral sex can transmit STIs.

Vaginal sex: Some people may only think of penile-vaginal sex as the standard definition here. However, vaginal sex can also involve inserting other objects into the vagina (such as a dildo or other sex toy) or vulva-to-vulva contact. Penile-vaginal sex can result in a pregnancy and/or transmission of STIs. Vulva-to-vulva sex can transmit STIs.

Anal sex: These are sex behaviors that involve inserting something into the anus—a penis, fingers, and/or sex toys. Anal sex can transmit STIs.

Sexually Transmitted Infections

Before your child chooses to enjoy sexual behavior, it's important that they understand the risks as well as the pleasures. Here are a few terms to help navigate the important health and safety conversations.

BACTERIAL STIs

Bacterial infections can be contracted from any skin-to-skin contact of the genitals or mouth. Kids need to know that penetration or intercourse are not necessary to be susceptible to sexually transmitted infection.

Chlamydia is a very common bacterial infection affecting about 3 million 14- to 24-year-olds each year. While often asymptomatic, symptoms can include pain/burning while peeing, belly pain, abnormal vaginal discharge (yellowish, strong smell), and bleeding between periods. Repeated, untreated infections can lead to problems in people assigned female, such as increased risk of pelvic inflammatory disease or ectopic pregnancy. It is spread by vaginal, anal, and oral sex—even without ejaculation—and can rarely be transmitted to the eyes by contact with fluid on hands.

Gonorrhea is a similarly common bacterial infection, most often affecting people in their teens and 20s. While often asymptomatic, symptoms can include pain/burning while peeing, belly pain, abnormal vaginal discharge (yellowish, strong smell), discharge in stools, rectal itching, and sores on the throat. Like chlamydia, untreated cases can cause health problems such as pelvic inflammatory disease. Also, the disease has been developing antimicrobial resistance, making prevention even more important. It is spread by vaginal, anal, and oral sex—even without ejaculation—and, rarely, can be transmitted to the eyes by contact with fluid on hands.

Syphilis is another bacterial infection that often goes unnoticed in its early stages. The first symptom is usually a small round sore, known as a chancre. It can develop on your genitals, anus, or mouth. Chancres are painless but very contagious. Further symptoms can include fever, fatigue, rash, headaches, joint pain, and weight and hair loss. If left untreated, late-stage syphilis can lead to loss of hearing, vision, or memory; mental illness; heart disease; infection of the brain or spinal cord; and death.

VIRAL STIs

The viral STIs have much greater consequences for a young person's sexual life because they stay in a body forever. Here is a brief list your daughter will need to be aware of:

Hepatitis B is a virus found in infected blood, semen, and vaginal fluid and can be transmitted through unprotected sex. You can also get it from contaminated needles and syringes. Symptoms include fever, fatigue, nausea, dark urine, and clay-colored bowel movements, among others.

Herpes Simplex Virus (HSV) is one of two main strains of the virus, HSV-1 and HSV-2. Both can be transmitted sexually. The CDC estimates more than 1 out of 6 people aged 14 to 49 in the United States have herpes. HSV-1 causes oral herpes, which is responsible for cold sores or blisters. However, it can also be passed from a person's mouth to another person's genitals during oral sex. HSV-2 primarily causes genital herpes sores to develop on or around the genitals.

Human Papillomavirus (HPV) is passed from one person to another through intimate skin-to-skin or sexual contact. There are many different strains of the virus. The most common symptom of HPV is **warts** on the genitals, mouth, or throat. Some strains can lead to cancer, including oral, vaginal, or anal, among others. HPV is the most common sexually transmitted infection among women. There is currently a highly effective vaccine available (Gardasil 9) that girls and boys can receive before becoming sexually active. More on that on page 41.

HIV is a virus that can be passed through anal or vaginal sex, intravenous drug use, and blood transfusion. It can damage the immune system and raise the risk of contracting other viruses or bacteria and developing certain cancers. If left untreated, HIV can lead to AIDS (Acquired Immuno-Deficiency Syndrome). But with pre-exposure prophylaxis (PrEP) as well as treatment after an HIV-positive diagnosis, many people living with HIV don't ever develop AIDS. In the early or acute stages, it's easy to mistake the symptoms of HIV with those of the flu. HIV is an important test for any STI screen before sexual activity.

Contraception

One of the biggest decisions your daughter may face is not whether to have sex, but when. A big part of that decision is protecting herself from infections or unplanned pregnancy. Here is an overview of terms to help guide that conversation.

External Condoms: Condoms are the only form of contraception that can reduce—but not completely eliminate—both the risk of STIs and pregnancy during sex. There is no minimum age to buy condoms. Help your daughter discover whether or not she has a latex allergy well before she is sexually active, so she can seek alternatives. It's important to remember that oil-based lubricants should never be used with latex condoms.

Internal Condoms: The internal condom is inserted into the vagina before sex to help prevent pregnancy. It can also reduce the risk of STIs. An internal condom can be inserted up to two hours before penile-vaginal intercourse and is only good for one use. An internal condom and an external condom should never be used at the same time as they can easily break from the friction.

Short-Term Contraception: The pill, **the patch**, **the ring**, and **the shot** are all hormonal options that can reduce the risk of pregnancy. These can allow an individual to have control over how often they get their period and can regulate the menstrual cycle. For the pill to be fully effective, a woman must take it every day at approximately the same time. So, it is best for a girl who is ready for that level of consistent routine and schedule. While rare, hormonal birth control has the potential to cause or exacerbate existing symptoms of mood disorders such as depression, so it is important to be aware of any extreme shifts in your daughter's mood.

Long-Term Contraception: An intrauterine device **(IUD)** may be inserted by a qualified health care provider into the uterus to prevent pregnancy. This option is available in hormonal form (also called **the rod**) or nonhormonal form, called Paragard, made of medical-grade copper, which can prevent pregnancy for up to 12 years.

Emergency Contraception: This is commonly known as **the morning-after pill**. The medication is taken after sex to reduce the risk of pregnancy if no protection was used or contraception failed. The brand Plan B can be purchased over the counter and does not have an age requirement. However, it must be taken within 72 hours of intercourse to be effective. Another brand, Ella, requires a prescription from a health care provider and can be taken up to 120 hours after sex; it is more effective for people weighing over 155 pounds. Both should be taken as soon as possible after intercourse or exchanging fluids with semen to be the most effective. Contrary to misconception, the morning-after pill does not cause an abortion; it prevents pregnancy by delaying ovulation or blocking implantation of a fertilized egg.

Abortion: Abortion is a simple health care intervention to end a pregnancy. Many people have strong feelings around abortion; be sure to talk to your daughter about your values around this topic. Two types of abortion are available: a medication abortion and a surgical abortion. A medication abortion involves taking pills prescribed by a doctor that will end a pregnancy. These pills are different from the morning-after pill mentioned on page 39. A surgical abortion involves a procedure that uses suction (called a D&C—dilation and curettage—similar to basic reproductive health procedures) to remove the fetus from the uterus. Laws governing how old a person needs to be, how advanced the pregnancy is, and whether a minor needs a parent's permission to have an abortion vary from state to state.

STI Treatment and Prevention

There are a handful of effective medications that can treat and/or prevent certain STIs. Antibiotics treat and cure chlamydia, gonorrhea, and syphilis. They also require a prescription from a health care provider.

In the 1980s, HIV and AIDS became a global pandemic, peaking in the early 1990s. Since then, medicine has evolved to create preventative options and encouraging long-term treatment.

Pre-exposure prophylaxis, also known as PrEP, is a daily medication (typically Truvada) that reduces a person's risk of acquiring HIV before they are exposed to it. PrEP is for sexually active people who may have a higher risk of acquiring HIV, and patients must get a prescription from a health care provider.

Post-exposure prophylaxis, also known as PEP, is a medication that can be taken up to 72 hours after sex to reduce the risk of acquiring HIV. The sooner PEP is taken after the sexual experience, the more effective it will be. Patients must get a prescription from a health care provider.

Gardasil 9 is a vaccine that helps protect individuals who are 9 to 45 years of age against the diseases caused by nine types of HPV. This includes cervical, vaginal, vulvar, and anal cancer, as well as certain throat and back-of-mouth cancers and genital warts. The Centers for Disease Control (CDC) currently recommends the HPV vaccine to young people ages 11–12. So, you may want to add this to your daughter's vaccine schedule before she becomes sexually active.

KEEP IN MIND

- Gender identity is the way a person experiences their core sense of self in regards to gender.
- Sexuality is our unique awareness, acceptance, and enjoyment of our own body and the bodies of others. Sexual orientation is about what causes us attraction, and who/what we desire in relationships.
- Pronouns matter; gender and sexual identity and expression can vary.
- There are many safe and healthy ways to enjoy pleasurable sex.

PART II

FOUNDATIONAL PARENTING STRATEGIES

In this section, we will take the wide view on parenting a girl today. These strategies provide a foundation for future conversations about any topic—including sexuality—helping to hone your message, build the necessary trust, and maintain open communication between you and your daughter.

The early adolescent years bring unique challenges in a society where young people live with their parents throughout puberty, their increasing independence, and beyond. Hopefully these guidelines will help you navigate the storms and shifts. Conversations about healthy sexuality, positive friendships, and personal development are all eventually connected, and they start by discovering your own values as a parent.

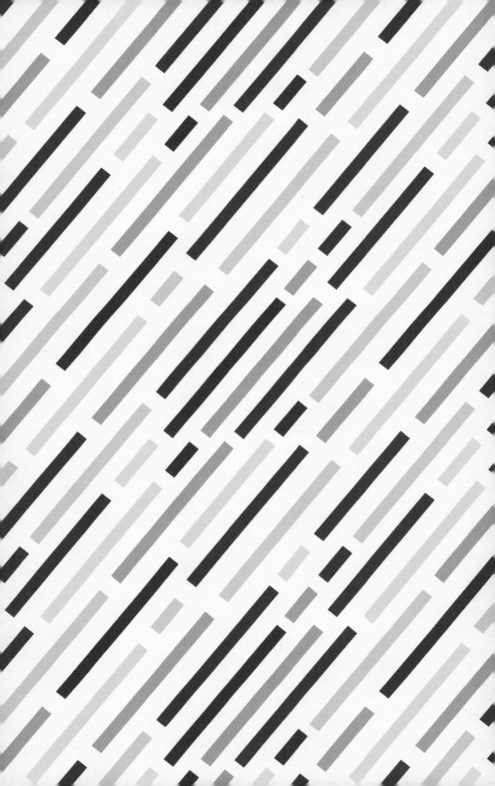

CHAPTER FOUR

Defining and Sharing Your Values

How do we discover what we value most? When I host sexuality education sessions for young people, I often start values conversations this way:

"Tell me about someone you really admire."

The young person talks about a person they hold in high regard. They share stories and moments that proved their worthiness of that elevated role in their eyes. Then, I reflect the **values** back to them.

For example, I remember one girl of about 12 sharing:

"My friend's mom is amazing. She had cancer last year, and she totally got through it. She was in bed for months, and my friend was so worried. Then, her mom showed up to our fundraiser and was smiling and selling cookies with us like it was the funnest thing she could ever imagine. She brought gifts for each of us, too. It's like, no matter what she's going through, she shows up and makes it a great experience for everyone."

I would reflect:

"I hear a value of resilience. *That when things are hard, she still finds a way to rise through it. Maybe also* generosity. *You admire how she continues to think of others and to give, no matter how much or little she has. Is there also a value of* joyfulness? *That you see her shining in enjoyment and you admire that about her, too . . ."*

The child nodded knowingly. This is one way to recognize our values. Inversely, our stories of anguish can often illuminate our values in reverse. If someone speaks often of betrayal, the value may be *loyalty*. If someone gets worked up about deceptions, the value is likely *honesty*.

Start now by listening for the **value** and the **need** in your own child's stories. You will be delighted by the relief this brings them, in hearing their core values reflected back.

Practical Guidelines

When I host "Raising Sexually Healthy Kids" seminars, adult participants often have revelations about their values around sex. I take them through the following exercise:

▶ Look over the following list and circle every value that positively speaks to you about sex. If it fills you with a "yes" and a sense of rightness, circle it. Add your own if it is not listed here. Circle about 10 to 12 if you get that far.

Safety	Privacy	Respect
Freedom	Boundaries	Encouragement
Connection	Consensual	Fun
Acceptance	Commitment-based	Devotion
Loyalty	Monogamy	Exploration
Family	Polyamory	Uninhibited

Communication	Attentiveness	Joyfulness
Comfort	Passion	Diverse (celebrating other orientations/ genders)
Humor	Presence	
Empathy	Honesty	Personal Growth
Intuition	Listening	Discovery
Spirituality	Openness	Pleasure
Sensuality	Friendship	Protection
Responsibility	Heart	
Fairness	Playfulness	Informed
Reverence	Love	Intimate

▶ Now, place an asterisk next to your top three values around sex.

▶ Once you've done this, answer the following question for yourself: *What is a key experience that shaped my perspective on sexuality and my holding of these values?*

▶ Now ask: *How might my values and experience influence my parenting of my daughter?*

Remember that influence is neither inherently negative nor positive—only informing of our views. Take time to consider the many ways this could play out for you as you guide your child around sex.

Here's another activity to try, as you clarify your values in anticipation of talking to your daughter about sex:

▶ Notice the conversations you share with loved ones over the course of one week. What is the emotion behind the story? What role do the characters involved play? What is your role?

▶ Now, notice the underlying theme—and identify the value or need. Sometimes the need (met or unmet) will direct us toward the value.

The best way we can support our daughters in healthy relationships and sex is to start reflecting a value or a need from her stories. Girls in particular are often socialized to ignore their own needs (and prioritize others'), so whenever you can help her articulate what she needs, it also adds a component of personal empowerment. "This is what you need" can be a powerful message to a girl going through puberty.

OPEN A DIALOGUE

To create emotional safety at home, we can be conscious of how we speak of others in their romantic and/or sexual experiences. We'll always be more effective imparting our values through comments on what we *appreciate* as opposed to sharing judgments. Every value you identified from the list can have an "I appreciated" expression.

If your value is **Equality**:

"Did you see how Thomas kept checking that Andrea was happy with their appetizer choice at the restaurant? He was so committed to making sure her preferences were taken into account. I really appreciate seeing that equality in couples."

If your value is **Safety**:

"So, Oscar stood up for Silas, even when the other men were picking on him? Wow. I really appreciate the courage it takes for partners to make sure everyone feels safe. So impressive."

The situations don't need to be inherently sexual or romantic, because the values will translate into her choice of partner in the future.

TAKEAWAYS

- Our values and needs reveal themselves in who we admire and in the stories we tell.
- Reflecting your daughter's values and needs gives her a sense of grounding and self-understanding—start this practice now.
- Remember, it's always okay to say to your daughter when talking about sex, "If I seem nervous when I'm talking about this, it's because it's totally new to me, and no one talked to me about it when I was a kid . . ."
- Reframe around your own values in parenting her: "I still want to talk because I care about the experiences you'll have with sex, and I want to be the one to support you . . ."
- Reinforce your values by naming what you appreciated about others in social situations when speaking to your daughter.

CHAPTER FIVE

Facilitating Openness

Connie Dawson and Jean Illsley Clarke share a poignant story in their book *Growing Up Again: Parenting Ourselves, Parenting Our Children*. This is one of my favorite stories about parents talking to kids about sex. Two 19-year-old daughters and their mothers take a long road trip for a girls vacation. From the back seat, a mother overhears her daughter say to her friend, "I wish my mom had told me that when I was younger." Excusing herself for the intrusion, the mother asks with curiosity, "What do you wish I had told you?" The daughter replies, "To wait until I was 18 to have sex."

"Really?!" the mother exclaims in utter surprise. The daughter continues, "I know, I would have rolled my eyes and said you were out of touch and clueless. But I needed someone else's voice in my ear, the voice of someone who loved me, when I stood toe-to-mushy-toe with a ninth-grade boy who told me I wanted to 'do it.'"

Sometimes, the moments of openness can seem elusive, especially during tense moments of resistance. Kids this age often test boundaries, push us away, challenge the strength of the connection, and evoke shouting matches. It can be understandably difficult to commit to maintaining openness. But, knowing all that an adolescent girl stands to gain can help us keep our focus and keep trying. Our daughters do hear us, even when outward signs may not show it.

Practical Guidelines

Here are a few basic guidelines to help keep communication open:

Empathize first, offer context/ guidance second

If our daughter comes to us with a situation in her life, it's best to offer her our support and understanding of *her* feelings first. If we begin with, "Well, they probably wanted to feel worthy," we run the risk of communicating loyalty to the other person, instead of supporting our daughter primarily. Our daughters will be more open with us when they sense that they are understood and accepted.

The puberty years will call for this even more. Self-consciousness and self-doubt are running high. So, to create a truly safe space, give a moment to just "be" compassionately with her in whatever she shares. Even breathing through a pause of, "Yeah, that must be hard . . ." puts her nervous system at ease. Then, give the guidance or context. "Sometimes, when people are jealous, they put others down to lift themselves up. Do you ever notice that?"

Address the emotion
beneath the behavior

If our limit of "You can't go to that party when no parents are home," is met with "You're the worst parent in the world!" it's important to simply pan back and see her pain. Try to avoid getting hung up on the hook of taunting or insults. Defending ourselves from that kind of emotional venting only escalates the conflict.

Try instead, "I see you're really angry about that. I know it will take some time to accept the disappointment that comes with my limit." Remember the power of tone here. The voice we use to correct our daughter now is likely the voice she will hear in her own mind when she corrects herself in the future.

Ask yourself, *If I were secure enough to not be affected by the slights, how could I respond?* It's not about their respect for us as a parent, or even as a human being. It's often an expression of their feeling safe enough to rage and discharge pent-up emotion.

Of course, we do have the right to set limits on their treatment of us. House rules like no name-calling, no profanity, etc., absolutely have a place. So, draw your own lines accordingly.

Appreciate the complexities
of individuation

Individuation, as described by Carl Jung, the Swiss founder of analytical psychology, is the process of "coming to selfhood" or "self-realization." For our daughters in sexual maturity, that means disconnecting from us enough to discover who they truly are. Simply put, individuation claims, "I am a separate me; I am not you."

Toddlers go through this as they recognize they are physically separate from their primary caregivers. Tweens and teens navigate individuation by recognizing they are separate socially and emotionally. Sometimes this means doing the opposite of what we suggest, just to claim selfhood. They must push away in order to take their place in the social world beyond the home.

Here are a few general guidelines for supporting healthy individuation:

- Let them have their selfhood, even when they assert it through moments of emotional meltdowns or defiance.
- Let them have their demonstrations of separateness within the bounds of health and safety (hair dyeing and ear piercing are some examples of potentially acceptable choices).
- Just focus on being their safe space, a secure home base, no matter what.
- Ask permission before offering feedback or guidance on their situation. "Would you like to hear my thoughts on the situation?"

A secure base for a child looks like this:

1. I am one with you.

2. I can leave you for a while.

3. I can come back, and you will be there.

We'll talk more about building mutual trust in the next chapter.

OPEN A DIALOGUE

Here are some statements to offer empathy and support her healthy individuation:

- "I see why you would feel that way."
- "That does sound really hard."
- "Of course you were disappointed."
- "You were so upset when that happened, naturally. Do you want my thoughts about the situation?"
- "You are really becoming your own person now."
- "I'm so amazed to learn about your unique thoughts and opinions."
- "You are like me in this way; you are unlike me in this way."
- "I know you get to choose who you become. I'm just lucky to get to be a part of it along the way."

Two Helpful Tools

It is especially important to keep the lines of communication open in the case of an emergency or unsafe social situations. For older teens (anyone who can drive or be driven by an older friend), I offer these two great tools for parents:

1. **The SOS "bail me out" code**—Talk with your daughter in advance and come up with a simple code she can text you that means "Please call me and say you need to come pick me up." One beauty of the prevalence of modern phones is the ability to ask for help discreetly and within seconds. Sometimes, teens will want to save face socially, yet need to leave a scene for their own comfort. Age can be a factor, as well. So, a simple "SOS" via text will let them answer your call and say, "Oh, hi Mom. Okay . . ." and tell her friends there is a family emergency, etc.

2. **The "no consequences conversation"**—A lot of pre-carious situations arise when drugs or alcohol are involved. In preparation, consider letting your daughter know—right now—that you give her the future blessing of a "no conse-quences conversation" if she ever needs help. A teen might long for their parent's support, yet choose to not reach out for fear of getting in trouble over alcohol, drugs, sneaking out, etc. If they have this pass, then you have the chance to help them when they may need it most.

TAKEAWAYS

- Empathize, empathize! It is the surest way to help her feel safe enough to share more and open up.
- Whenever possible, let the angry outbursts roll off your back—and speak only to what she must be feeling.
- Reinforcing our daughter's separateness as an individual can actually help her feel freer to be open with us.
- Even when we don't truly "get it," we can always show her acceptance and nonjudgment.
- When correcting her, use a tone of voice that communi-cates total encouragement of who she is becoming.
- Plan a simple SOS signal to pick her up from unsafe social situations.
- Offer her the "no consequences conversation."

CHAPTER SIX

Establishing Mutual Trust

12-year-old Tianna storms into the house after school and throws her bag at the bottom of the stairs. The contents go flying. Her mother, Elise, walks in to find this and says, "Please put your bag in your room." Tianna roars, "Why can't I ever just have peace? It's always 'Do this!', 'Be more!', 'Be better!' I can't take it anymore!" Elise chooses to let go of the poor treatment of home and belongings (for now). She takes a deep breath and says gently, "What happened that makes you feel you don't have peace in being enough?"

Tianna quips a few "Nothing" remarks while she repacks her bag. Elise remains calmly present. She has the energy that day. Elise asks, "Was it something somebody said today?" A moment of resistance flashes across Tianna's face. Then, she crumples into sobs, "The teacher asked this question at book group—and I knew the answer—but Aidan raised his hand first, and then the teacher made this comment about how our group needed to be more prepared. Grrr!"

"So, it felt unfair to you because you never had the chance to show what you knew?" Elise offers. Tianna nods angrily, but with relief. "Just because Aidan is fast and loud in class doesn't mean we weren't prepared! Everyone in our group felt so bad, and I can't be everything." "Nobody can," Elise confirms. Tianna continues, "I always thought of myself as the smart one, but now it's like I don't know . . ."

Elise stays with Tianna a few extra minutes while she breathes more slowly and offers her reassurance. Once things are fully calm, Elise concludes, "It can be really hard to question who you are in a group setting like that. I know you'll always find a way to trust your own intelligence, regardless of what a teacher says." Tianna feels reassured. Elise smiles a bit—sensing the shift—and says, "Let's just not take it out on your backpack next time." Tianna returns a slightly embarrassed laugh and agrees. "Okay."

If Elise had remained focused on Tianna's behavior, she would have missed a rich opportunity to guide her daughter through a moment of personal doubt. The limit-setting came at the end, after her child felt total reassurance and acceptance. While this isn't always available in parenting moments, it is possible. Elise created trust by staying steady in the storm and being consistent on limits after first reassuring her.

Remember, only one person (ideally) is having their entire sense of self untethered and remade while their body changes beyond their control: our child.

Practical Guidelines

One way to think of trust between two people is a series of unanswered questions whose truths are revealed over time. If the emotional displays we're witnessing tell us something about our daughter's uncertainty now, what is the unaddressed question?

Will you still accept me when I am filled with rage?

What if I become withdrawn and sad?

Will you still keep me safe when I feel out of control?

How will I be safe in the world without relying on your protection?

All kinds of unanswered questions can arise for our girls in puberty, often without our realizing. They are likely testing out new identities among their peers at school. At home, there is an even more vital question: *Will my parent or primary caretaker accept me as I explore this part of who I am? Will they stay present when this new intensity of emotion throws me off center?*

So, how do we develop the strength to stay lovingly present during our teen's emotional meltdowns? What if the conflict is not truly between us as parent and child, but rather, as a parent and a child discharging stress in a space that feels safe?

Learn to Downshift When Tempers Run High

As Drs. Laura Kastner and Jennifer Wyatt write in *Getting to Calm: Cool-Headed Strategies for Parenting Tweens + Teens*, "Even if teens instigate an argument, grown-ups are responsible for bringing it to a halt." Sometimes, our child will goad us and provoke a fight in order to engage and work through intense feelings. Depending on temperament, a parent's voice can quickly become shrill or booming and intimidating.

Listen for the emotional pitch and tempo of your own voice. Sometimes, we're so tuned in to our kids that we don't realize we are following their emotional lead. Choose to not match your daughter's tone, but shift to a lower speed and tempo. When your daughter revs up the intensity, you can remain absolutely present while choosing consciously to mismatch the emotional tone.

OPEN A DIALOGUE

Things can get heated quickly during the teen years. Our fears for their safety peak to new heights, and their need for independence brings new levels of agitation. How can we stay present and reinforce trust?

"I'm feeling overwhelmed, and I want to be able to speak calmly with you about this. I'm going to take five minutes to catch my breath and meet you back here after I've cooled down."

"I don't know what to say right now, but I want you to know I care. Even when I am confused or frustrated, I am always caring about you."

"This is really hard for both of us. Let's just breathe together until we can talk in a better way about this."

Check your own heart rate and breathing, and make sure you're taking good care of your body. Try not to have important discussions when anyone is thirsty, hungry, or needs to pee. As the parent, you can call a moment's pause to make sure needs are met before proceeding. Whether it's a quick break to tend to your breathing, reframe unhelpful thoughts, or address your physical needs, a few minutes to regroup and resume can make all the difference.

Affirm the Feeling, Redirect the Behavior

As during the toddler years, we now have the chance to help our daughters trust themselves and still be safe in the world. Now, of course, we are referring to the much larger world they are gradually entering.

When our daughter tries out a certain defiance or disruptive choice, we can address the feeling while correcting the behavior. The message is simply, "*Yes* to what you are going through inside. *No* to what you're currently doing with it." We're all learning how to best manage internal desires, frustrations, longings, and emotions.

Sometimes, we may need to make a guess at the emotion beneath the behavior. "Okay, I see you're really angry right now . . ." This can be met with a fierce, "I'm not angry, I'm frustrated with you!" Here, we both get it wrong and become the momentary focus of their distress. An open-ended question is the best recovery here: "What is going on for you right now?" Remember that "what" and "how" questions are always more effective than "why" questions.

A safer affirmation can be, "Wow, you're really struggling with this . . ." in a tone of honest observation. Regardless of whether we may think the situation warrants a different reaction, we are not going through it. Often, these are multi-layered experiences. Just validating her struggle can be incredibly useful.

TAKEAWAYS

- Holding consistency in our limits builds trust with our daughters.
- Renegotiate any new limits at a later time, together (not on the fly).
- Address deeper, underlying uncertainties with proactive reassurance.
- We can accept their inner experience while correcting for behavior.
- Increase your "staying power" in heated moments by consciously mismatching an alarmed tone with a lower, more grounded voice.
- Just breathing through an unknown or difficult moment together can greatly increase trust.
- Even when they rail against our limits, consistency is what they need.

CHAPTER SEVEN

Respecting Boundaries

Boundaries affirm our selfhood and help us know where we truly stand in the world. Many a "nice" person finds themselves confused when things go awry after their failure to be clear on boundaries. While all genders can struggle with setting clear boundaries, girls in particular are conditioned in our culture to be people-pleasers and to put others' needs and desires before their own. The consequences of this behavior in sexual relationships could be quite devastating.

A healthy relationship to boundaries is a profound gift we can give our daughters at any age. Simply put, this means honoring her limits and teaching her to honor and accept her own. Increasing her awareness of boundaries in the early puberty years can reinforce healthy relationship lessons outside the home. This gives her a solid foundation for an empowered relationship to sex when she chooses to become sexually active.

Practical Guidelines

The inner work of boundaries is clarifying our personal lines of what is acceptable and not acceptable. The outer work is speaking and defending that truth with others. Boundaries are authentic and healthy when our self-love rises up to meet our "no." The realization comes from within and is bolstered by our inner love and acceptance moving outward. When we think that all the love and acceptance exists "out there" (as bestowed by others), it becomes harder to uphold a boundary.

The primary reason people fail to defend their boundaries is a fear of losing connection. Other reasons include:

- Wanting to avoid criticisms they have witnessed about "party-poopers" or "wet-blankets" (insert generationally appropriate put-down here).
- Lack of belief in their right to have limits or to speak up for them.
- Detachment from inner knowing because of early abuse, trauma, or a simple lack of personal reflection.
- Individual or group punishment for asserting oneself.

Your unique subculture likely determines which social messaging most contributes to any challenge your daughter could meet in learning boundaries. For some people, it can become a safety issue. Disparities in racial, financial, and other privileges directly inform the realities some face.

Yet, within our chosen intimate relationships, clear boundaries are crucial to health. This is a muscle most tweens and teens need to build during these years. We sometimes watch our teen make concessions in order to feel safe and enjoy (superficial) belonging, much to our pain and frustration. Remind her that being honest about her limits is a gift—and misleading people is no favor to anyone involved, herself included.

Define Who Is Responsible for What

It is said that people with boundary confusion tend to be overly responsible for others and under-responsible for themselves. How does this look in a teen's life?

Under-responsible	"Kayla made me so mad today! She was cheating off my test, and she should know that's not okay. It totally ruined my day, and it's all her fault."	someone else controls their emotions; the other person should somehow register and respond to the unspoken boundary; giving away power
Responsible	"I was so mad when Kayla tried to cheat off my math test today. I was just shocked that she would even think that was okay! I had to pull her aside after class and tell her I don't ever cheat—even when my friends forgot to study."	owning one's feelings as theirs; takes action to communicate personal boundary; stays empowered
Over-responsible	"Oh, poor Kayla had a huge fight with her older brother last night and was up crying until 2 a.m. I want to make it better. She didn't have time to study for the math test. I can fix this by letting her copy my work, just this one time . . ."	feels obligated to tend to situations they did not create; yields on personal stance or principles; considers "niceness" a supreme virtue above self-respect

Model Healthy Boundaries

Our daughters learn most powerfully by watching how we assert and respect our own boundaries. Letting her see us defend personal boundaries with friends, colleagues, partners, parents, or neighbors is a valuable teaching tool. If our child is not present at the time, and you want to encourage healthy boundaries for your girl, you can still share these stories with her throughout the week.

This witnessing also includes her seeing us set limits on how we let her treat us during arguments. For healthy modeling, consider this:

"Look, I understand you are really upset right now, but you are not allowed to speak to me like that. We have a family rule of no name-calling. I wouldn't want anyone talking to you that way, and I can't let you talk to me that way either."

This also reflects the boundary of disengagement. Sometimes, gracefully removing ourselves from a situation when things are heated is the most loving, self-respecting response. She may need to do the same at some point in the future.

If our child attempts to put extra pressure on us to "fix" a situation beyond anyone's reasonable control, or we find our own systems going into overload, it's best to disengage briefly. In an especially tense situation, it can be helpful to say something like "I know there don't seem to be any good solutions right now," and then telling your daughter you're going to make some tea and come back in 20 minutes to revisit the issue.

This time lets a child calm their systems without wrangling a parent down with them. They need accompaniment or witnessing, but not a fellow mate with whom to spiral into the abyss. When we come back, a clear and calm resolution is much more possible.

We'll talk more about consent (and tea) in chapter 16 (page 114).

OPEN A DIALOGUE

Sometimes, setting boundaries can be a challenge. Help your daughter become familiar with simple language to assert a boundary so she has it available in all kinds of situations: simple requests, peer pressure, and (eventually) sex . . .

- "This is not okay with me."
- "I am not comfortable with that."
- "I can't do that today."
- "I'm going to pass."
- "That doesn't work for me."
- "I need some time to think about that."
- "Let me get back to you on this."
- "No, thank you."
- "Nope."
- "No."
- "Not a fit."
- "That's out of line."
- "I can't accept that."
- "I'd rather do something else."
- "That's not going to work."
- "I need to make another choice."
- "Thanks for asking, but I'll say no."
- "Not for me."

TAKEAWAYS

- We can teach boundaries in conversation, reflection, and modeling.
- Encourage your daughter to ask herself, *Which of my relationships allow me to easily set boundaries?*
- Learning to set boundaries in the teen years is an ongoing strengthening practice.
- Teach her how to take appropriate responsibility—but not too much.
- Self-love upholds our boundaries—and supports rejection resilience.
- Accepting someone else's "no" is just as important as learning to defend hers.

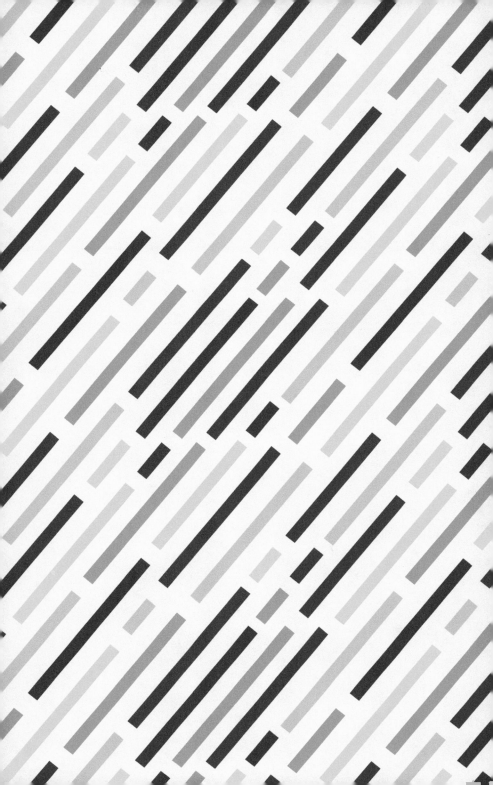

PART III

SPECIFIC
SEXUAL
HEALTH
STRATEGIES
FOR GIRLS

It's time to start applying these concepts directly to guiding our daughters around sexuality. Whether they are still young, just entering puberty, or well into adolescence, you can begin laying the strongest foundation as soon as possible.

If thinking of your daughter as a sexual being is still a distant or intimidating concept at this point, try holding these strategies as tools for helping her become a remarkable young woman overall.

Don't worry about being "too late," because a helpful message holds the power to steer us toward better experiences at any stage of life.

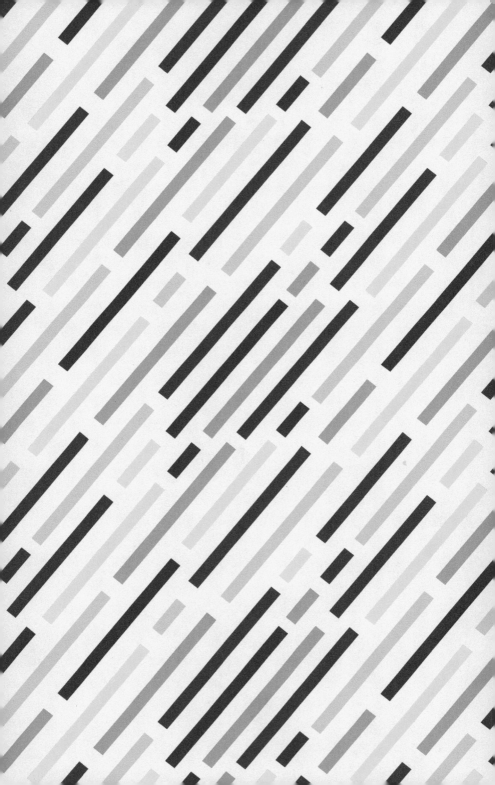

CHAPTER EIGHT

Preparing for Periods

The first menstrual cycle (menarche) is a significant moment in the life of many women. I have seen firsthand how this biological rite of passage for many women can shape their sense of power and comfort in their own bodies for decades. Some of us have embarrassing stories of getting our first period, some of us started with little information or support, and the lucky among us were informed and prepared. For a few, our first period was even celebrated as our sacred entry into womanhood.

Whether your daughter has begun menstruating or not, these guidelines will still greatly support her healthy experience of her body. Even a transgender child who may or may not menstruate will benefit from understanding the process and how to support it. When it comes to lovingly encouraging the body, it's rarely ever too late.

Practical Guidelines

The menstrual cycle has natural phases, just like the day, the year, and the seasons. When people begin menstruating, they embody this wisdom more deeply. The first day of bleeding is considered day 1. From days 1 to 14, between menstruation and ovulation (the release of the egg from the ovary), the cycle may bring a surge of positive energy. The menstruating person may notice feeling more outgoing, active, and engaged with the world.

From days 15 to 28 (or, ovulation onward), the menstruating person naturally experiences a downshift in energy and a drawing inward. This counterbalance is highly health-enhancing, even as we live in a culture that favors extraversion, activity, and outward appearances. When you are speaking to your child about menstruation, consider reframing the second half of the cycle—the days before menstruation—as a guidepost to listen to and heed the body's deeper wisdom. This may feel countercultural to some. Yet, many of the negative physical symptoms of PMS (premenstrual syndrome) are signs that the body needs replenishment, quiet, and/or emotional tending and release.

For some, the natural ebb and flow of energy with the menstrual cycle becomes difficult to manage for physiological reasons. Unwelcome mood changes, increased irritability, anxiety, and sadness can arise, and these need to be met with patience and compassion. While rare, some women also experience a more severe condition called premenstrual dysphoric disorder (PMDD), which can greatly disrupt one's life. It affects up to 5 percent of women of childbearing age and warrants medical assistance. If your daughter's mood changes are so severe that they're interfering with school and relationships, or you are worried about her mental health, it is a good idea to talk with your doctor. Other conditions such as endometriosis can present as painful periods. So, seek help whenever you have questions.

Pain Management

For many girls and women, the time before and during menstruation brings minor physical discomfort such as bloating, weight gain, headaches, breast tenderness, acne flare-ups, fatigue, joint or muscle soreness, and cramps. The cause of cramps is the subtle contraction of the muscles lining the uterus. The body is drawing fluid from the entire system to flush and shed the lining, so staying thoroughly hydrated prevents many of the discomforts of cramping. Most cases of cramps can be eased with rest, a hot water bottle, or a warm bath, but for more severe pain, ibuprofen can help.

OPEN A DIALOGUE

What does your daughter think about periods? You may not know unless you ask. Negative, outdated advertising may be behind us now, but she is likely forming opinions about menstruation in unexpected ways.

Before your daughter reaches age 10 (or anytime!), try inviting an open-ended discussion about menstruation and see what unfolds.

"What have you heard about periods?"

"Do you have any friends who have started, and what do they say?"

"What kinds of things can you do when you are menstruating? What can't you do?"

"Can you think of anything positive about the experience?"

Kids can reach some surprising conclusions in the absence of practical information. Start the demystification together now.

The Period Bag

Knowing what to expect physically is a great source of assurance for kids who will menstruate, and having a period bag ready is a powerful tool to ease their tension. This is a pouch to hold supplies a person will need during their period. It can be simple and home-made, using a pencil case or cloth toiletry bag—or you can buy designer ones with a hook to hang the bag vertically in a bathroom stall while your child accesses what they need.

It can include:

- reusable cloth or disposable pads of varying sizes
- damp wipes in individual packages
- a change of underwear
- a waterproof pouch or zip-top bag to hold used items

Menstruation Care Options

There are several options on the market to absorb menstrual flow (probably more than when you were a kid). Being educated about what's available, and the pros and cons of each option, will help your daughter choose what's right for her.

Menstrual Pads. These days, reusable cloth pads are just as comfortable and accessible as disposable—with added environmental and cost benefits. If your daughter chooses disposable pads during her period, make sure she understands that they cannot be flushed down any toilet. They need to be wrapped on themselves or in tissue and disposed of (away from pets who may be drawn to the fluid).

Tampons are dense bundles of absorbent cotton inserted into the vagina. They are more discreet and sometimes preferred during certain athletic activities. But they require special instructions—and carry unique risks. Girls will need to understand toxic shock syndrome and how to use tampons responsibly. I recommend starting younger girls with pads and revisiting this option later, once they have some comfort and experience.

The Diva Cup is a reusable medical-grade silicone cup inserted into the vagina that collects and holds menstrual fluid until it is ready to be emptied and reinserted. A girl will need to be willing to handle it in public restrooms and keep it clean.

Period Underwear is the latest development in reusable menstrual supplies—and many companies have created seamless alternatives.

Acknowledging the Transition

I encourage parents to find a way to acknowledge this profound transition in a way that is meaningful for their family—one that supports and honors their daughter in a way she is comfortable with. This could be something simple and private like a spa day with mom or a hike or special dinner with the family, or you can host a rite of passage ceremony like a Red Party that involves your wider community (see the Resources section [page 138]). Every family— and every girl—is different, so choose what feels appropriate to celebrate your daughter's arrival into this new phase of life.

TAKEAWAYS

- Share what you can about the positive power of menstruation, or ask the women in your life to share insights with your menstruating daughter.
- Charting her cycle through waking temperature, mucus changes, and mood can empower a girl to truly know her body (See Resources, page 138).
- Offer her a range of menstrual supply options and instructions.
- Acknowledge and honor this profound transition by celebrating this new phase of life in your own way.

CHAPTER NINE

Combating Negative Body Image

Andrew and Lillian were very conscious of raising a healthy, empowered girl. They ate well, had an active lifestyle, and were aware of how they spoke about other people's bodies. Still, Andrew reported to me, "We work so hard to say only positive things about her body, about our bodies . . . Then, Rosa starts gymnastics at nine years old, and comes home and says, 'I'm fat.' We cried."

Andrew and Lillian went to the gymnastics instructors to talk about what was happening in class for their nine-year-old. "Rosa said the teacher told her that the girls needed to 'tuck in their bellies' whenever they were up on the balance beam," they told the gym's director. "It's causing problems in how the girls see their bodies." The gym's owners were embarrassed and apologetic, and they did what they could to address the language used about bodies. But ultimately, Lillian and Andrew decided to take Rosa out of gymnastics.

Don't be surprised if you do everything you can think of to be a body-positive and encouraging family—and still find yourself facing this issue. We can do everything we can to protect our daughters from unhealthy messaging about female bodies, but they will still be exposed to it somehow, whether through activities like Rosa's gymnastics, in movies and TV shows, in magazines, on social media, in advertising, at school, or through friends.

It is not a natural instinct for girls to look at their bodies and declare, "Wrong!" It is—as they say about systemic injustice at the Racial Equity Institute—"something in the groundwater."

According to the South Carolina Department of Mental Health, it is estimated that over 8 million Americans have an eating disorder (7 million women, 1 million men). The American Academy of Child and Adolescent Psychiatry suggests that as many as 1 in every 10 girls suffers from an eating disorder, the most common being anorexia nervosa, bulimia, and bingeing disorder. This does not even take into account more subtle forms of disordered eating like constant dieting, nor the insidious effects of having an unloving relationship with their bodies.

Practical Guidelines

How can we combat these realities as parents?

First, let your daughter know that misrepresentation of bodies is a much larger social problem. For example, in June 2021, it became illegal in Norway for social media influencers to share photos of their body that have been retouched without labeling them as edited. Most of the airbrushed and Photoshopped actors, musicians, influencers, and other entertainers your daughter sees in mainstream entertainment are not representative of what real, normal people actually look like. Part of what entertainment does is sell a fantasy, and that includes a fantasy of what people—especially women—look like.

As mentioned before, teens of all genders tend to suffer from a kind of overfocus on the self and a "fishbowl" perception. They think everyone is looking at them and seeing all their flaws. They are naturally hyperaware, so, you can offer a new perspective by placing her experience into the larger struggle for healthy female representation.

Media Literacy

The way you respond to media is a tool to teach your child about sex, your values, and healthy choices. This also clearly applies to body image. Tweens and teens with access to social media are enjoying the rush of believing they now have direct access to the larger world—only, it is a distorted world. So, what can we say to balance the allure of such seeming freedoms?

Media literacy is the ability to critically assess what we see in popular media through a practical lens of health. Even though it may annoy your daughter, feel free to point out often when something is clearly fake, airbrushed, or even unrealistic.

Celebrate "real" bodies wherever you can. Start looking for opportunities to offer a lens through which to see that *real is beautiful*. Adolescents still have a hard time distinguishing fantasy from reality, so we need a message that helps them dispel the myth of body perfection.

OPEN A DIALOGUE

We have a great opportunity when our daughters ask us, "How do I look?" Try a response that speaks to her experience of her body:
- "You look really delighted in that outfit."
- "You look a little uncertain or restricted."
- "You seem comfortable and confident in that one."
- "How do you feel?"

Reframe Attractiveness

Years ago, I trained as a facilitator in Teen Talking Circles with Linda Wolf, who had been organizing honest sharing circles among teen girls and boys for years. She revealed something powerful, in relation to heterosexuality and attraction.

She asked a group of heterosexual boys:

What is most attractive to you in a girl?

The answers were written anonymously on slips of paper. When Wolf shared the responses with the group of girls, they were surprised by them. The girls expected them to be all about thinness or prettiness. The top answer by a landslide fit one common theme:

When a girl is really excited about something she's into.

Imagine that—being energized by a personal passion makes us more attractive to others!

Often beneath the longing to "look right" is the deeper desire for acceptance and loving connection in a romantic/sexual partner. This is highly useful for us as parents because it allows us to potentially address the deeper concern—and take the focus off the finer details of the body (as it changes).

Thinking beyond the initial attraction, we can bring a refreshing perspective here as well. What draws us to people over time? What keeps love alive and relationships close?

Tell your daughter that, while looks might attract initially, it is the quality of our inner character strengths and traits in action that sustain love. These play a larger role in how we see someone's attractiveness over time.

Stay Aware of Her Eating Habits and Speak Up If Concerned

The solution to an acute eating disorder can be a real investment of time, medical care, and psychological support. If your daughter shows signs of being secretive about food, limiting her intake unnecessarily, or begins to look malnourished despite your best efforts, talk to your doctor. Early intervention is key to a strong recovery.

Please also see the Resources section (page 138) for more information.

TAKEAWAYS

- Teach your daughter media literacy—how to challenge unrealistic images of girls' and women's bodies—and offer alternatives.
- Comment on body portrayal in the media and celebrate those that highlight realistic and diverse bodies.
- Tell her that the real beauty of our bodies is how we enjoy and experience them.
- Reassure her about the deeper need for love, acceptance, and connection—that physical details are not what sustain love.
- Begin celebrating the joyful embodiment of women of all shapes and sizes in your day-to-day language.

CHAPTER TEN

Nurturing Self-Worth and Self-Respect

Carrie Ann, a 39-year-old mother, shares the story of a time when her eight-year-old daughter, Dimitri, mimicked what she saw—and it brought Carrie Ann to a halt. She recalls, "Dimitri spilled milk while pouring a very tall glass for the first time. She threw up her hands and shouted, 'Agh, I'm so clumsy and stupid!' I recoiled from watching her say that about herself . . . Then, I remembered I had just spilled the rice while serving dinner earlier that week and said the very same thing! I didn't even realize she'd heard me say that."

For Carrie Ann, it was a wake-up call to the power of modeling and our own self-worth and self-respect. She is now more conscious of her own self-talk and has started saying things like "Darn, I would have liked to handle that better," or "Okay, I'm really struggling right now—but I've got this," when she messes up.

How do we talk to ourselves when things are hard? When we mess up, make mistakes, or experience failure? Does our daughter hear us beat ourselves up, or is it compassion, acceptance, and resilience that we demonstrate?

Confidence can be relatively easy for most of us when things are golden. When we (or life circumstances) falter, we have an opportunity to show our girls what it means to hold ourselves well.

Practical Guidelines

One of the most powerful things we can teach our daughters is to stop apologizing for taking up space. Girls and women are taught to say "sorry" and play small as a way to momentarily feel safe or be "likable." This may be an especially significant issue for Black women, women of color, disabled women, tall women, and fat women. Anyone who receives social messaging that they are less valued in the world may unconsciously recoil or stoop when moving among people in public.

Let's show our girls the power of moving confidently and without apology. Training in body language can go a long way here—your daughter has likely heard you tell her to stand up straight. Try to also tell her to look forward, make eye contact, and be clear about her right to be on this planet.

I often observe this unhelpful "over-apologizing" tendency in women who say "sorry" when they pass others in a small space or need to get by. Are we truly sorry? Being in that space was not a violation. It is two people navigating a sidewalk or the aisle at the grocery store. For years now, I've been consistently responding with "Don't be sorry," essentially as a public service announcement. Attention: you have nothing to be sorry for!

Accepting Compliments

It is a sign of maturity and self-respect when someone can graciously receive a compliment. Help your daughter watch for any tendency to "deny" positive things said about her. One who stays steady and replies simply, "Thank you for the compliment," is showing a measure of personal power.

I've heard it said that true confidence is a state of being unaffected by either criticism or praise—meaning that we know our value truly, without crumbling under critique or seeking (or growing embarrassed) by praise.

Statements like . . .

"Oh, no, I'm not that smart/pretty/etc."

"It's just a little thing," (in reference to a gesture of generosity or accomplishment).

"I've been really blessed," (when referring to something that took real effort to achieve).

. . . all undermine a girl's confidence. While they may be common socially, they are not normal or necessary.

"You did really well on that music performance last night," need only be met with a strong and steady, "Thank you."

Sometimes, we can all forget how far we've come. Helping girls see how they are better—even this week compared to last week—nurtures self-worth by affirming their growth.

For example:

"Last week, you were really stressed-out because you kept choosing to play video games instead of studying. I noticed that this week, you stopped much earlier and had a far better time at school. Congratulations on finding the discipline to do that—I know it takes strength, and you really found your focus."

Here, we are affirming true progress on a layered skill: personal discipline, focus, and strength. She can own these as true *because she lived them in action* and will likely build on them from here.

The Power of an Apology

Apologies are a positive sign of healthy self-worth and respect. They heal fractures and allow trust to return after difficult moments.

On one end of the spectrum are those who simply do not apologize. They tend to blame or criticize others but never own up in a balanced way (e.g., "I'm sorry you feel that way").

As parents, we can instead give our daughters a "you are worth my apology" message. Even if we don't meet our own standards for how we want to react to our kids, we can always give them the message that the standard is there to be met. It's about what they deserve. When we fall short, we can offer:

"I feel really badly about how I spoke to you earlier today. I was overwhelmed by a hard day at work, and my tone had nothing to do with you. I did not keep my voice calm—and I'm sorry for that."

I know that some of you may have a reflexive jerking back. You need to stay in control as the parent, right?

The truth is, we will all often have moments when we need to apologize to our daughters. Here, we have an opportunity to demonstrate a healthy, balanced self-respect—while communicating to them that they deserve better treatment than we were able to give in that moment.

Template for a great apology:

1. "I'm sorry I . . ." (specific action or choice made)

2. "Here's what was going on for me inside . . ." (vulnerable sharing)

3. "I recognize it caused you pain," or "How did that affect you?"

4. "I want to do better. I will . . ." (specific course correction) and/or "What do you need from me now?"

5. "How can I make things right?"

TAKEAWAYS

- Give your daughter heartfelt apologies that convey your respect for her.
- Teach her to avoid over-apologizing for commonplace things—"Excuse me" is often more appropriate than a reflexive "Sorry" in public spaces.
- Show her how to graciously accept a compliment (without self-diminishment).
- Reflect the details of her progress on character traits and growth over time.
- Consider that cultivating the "internal locus" of self-respect is more enduring than looking to the outside world for validation.

CHAPTER ELEVEN

Discussing Masturbation and Pleasure

Aisha, now in her late 20s, did not receive the kind of sex education most of us would want for our daughters. Her family did not talk about sex, and she received an abstinence-only curriculum in her small-town public school, which only provided information about the basic mechanics of procreation. She was never taught about the function of the clitoris (100 percent for pleasure) or that women could even have orgasms. When she started having sex with her boyfriend in her late teens, she couldn't figure out what all the fuss was about. It seemed to her that boys were the only ones really enjoying sex.

It wasn't until Aisha was in college, hearing female friends talk about what they enjoyed in sex that she realized how much she'd been missing. No one had ever taught her the functions and power of her own anatomy, let alone having a right to sexual pleasure. She had grown up so distanced from her own body that she'd never felt free to explore it through masturbation. She had no idea what to ask for from her sexual partners because she had never given herself the space to discover what she wanted in the first place.

Aisha was angry. She felt cheated. But more than that, she was determined to make it right, to give her body the pleasure—and the respect—it deserved. She made it her mission to educate herself, and she vowed that if she ever had a daughter, she would not make the same mistakes her parents did.

Unfortunately, Aisha's story is not an uncommon one. We live in a culture that is obsessed with sex, but also terrified to talk about it in an honest and open way—especially with our daughters. But as parents and caregivers, we have the power to break that cycle and empower our girls to grow up secure in knowing they have the right to pleasure. This includes sharing basic information they need to discover what pleasure means for them.

So, how exactly do we do that?

Practical Guidelines

First, teach your daughter the intricacies of her own anatomy. Let's start with the basics. The external genitalia of most people assigned female can be distinguished by the clitoris, labia, vaginal opening, and opening to the urethra (for urine). It can be a revelation to young girls (and some adults) that people assigned female have three holes between their legs: the opening to the urethra, the opening to the vagina, and the anus.

Again, the whole of the sexual anatomy is not the vagina. The **vagina** is the interior canal between the vaginal opening and cervix that cannot be seen from the outside. The outer, fleshy folks we see are called the **labia majora**. The inner folds, which are unique to each body and often grow just beyond the labia majora at puberty, are called the **labia minora** (similar to the Spanish word for "lips"). **Vulva** refers to the outer, visible parts—the clitoris, labia, vaginal opening, and opening to the urethra.

The Clitoris

If she is eight or older, I can assure you it is okay to tell your daughter about the bundle of nerves at the top of the labia called the clitoris. The external nub, or *glans clitoris*, is above the opening to the urethra (in the middle) and the opening to the vagina (below). Its sole purpose is pleasure. The equivalent in those with a penis and testes is the head or glans of the penis. The clitoris has at least 8,000 nerve endings—with a glans and a "hood," much like a foreskin on an uncircumcised penis. It can (like a penis) become erect, swells in size when stimulated, and is the peak of sensation. The internal portions of the clitoris divide into two "roots" that wrap around the urethra and extend to the top of the vagina. The fabled G-spot is considered by many researchers to be part of this clitoral network, an area where internal clitoral nerve endings are more concentrated near the vaginal wall.

Our daughters need to know about the clitoris!

If your child is intersex (born with genitalia that does not neatly fit into the male/female binary) or transgender, this point will hold a different relevance, as sexual anatomy has many parallel and related features in all bodies. Recognizing this will help kids of all shapes and genders to feel empowered. Many women would also urge me here to ask you to teach your children assigned male at birth about the clitoris, as well (their future partners will thank you!).

Being intricately informed about the body's organs, their functions, and their accurate names is a great asset to mental and physical health. This knowledge gives a sense of agency, control, and power as kids grow through the disruptive years of puberty. When we know our bodies well, we can love them better.

Masturbation Is Healthy

No one can say with absolute certainty what someone will do with relevant information about their body—except (I would assert) feel more confident living in it. Kids may discover masturbation spontaneously as young as four or five years old. A very young body can orgasm (the rapid muscle contractions that release tension and bring pleasure); a person with a penis and testes will simply not ejaculate until sometime during puberty. A person with a vagina and ovaries can also ejaculate fluid through the paraurethral glands at the opening of the urethra when sexually aroused.

I have a colleague in sexual health—an MD with extensive training—whose primary messaging on masturbation to her daughters is, "Just make sure your hands are clean." Because the opening of the vagina leads to the internal organs of the cervix and uterus, clean hands are important. It's pretty simple. This kind of acceptance helps our daughters flourish.

If we want our daughters to enjoy their sexual experiences at some point, we have to allow them the freedom to explore their own bodies. Imagine how much more confident *any* young person would feel going into their first sexual experiences with an understanding of their own preferences and physiological responses. It's the difference between bringing your own map and just hoping your traveling companion knows where you are going.

Health benefits of masturbation include:

- better sleep
- reduced stress
- increased serotonin and dopamine levels—creating greater happiness
- oxygenation of the brain and improved mental clarity
- teaching girls what they like so they can be empowered to communicate it to a partner later in life
- increased confidence
- easing menstrual cramps by strengthening pelvic muscles

If masturbation becomes compulsive (interferes with regular activities) or you have concerns, see chapter 12 (page 92).

OPEN A DIALOGUE

While it may feel awkward to bring it up, many a young adult can be spared unnecessary self-doubt by knowing masturbation is healthy and normal. You are the safest person for them to hear it from.

During conversations about anatomy (age 8 to 10), try:

"Your clitoris is the bundle of nerves at the top of your labia. It feels good when you touch it—and it's okay to explore that feeling by yourself and in private."

About body diversity and acceptance (age 9 to 11):

"Different kinds of touch feel good for different bodies. You can discover what feels good to you when you're by yourself."

For girls age 10 to 12 (or sooner!):

"Our bodies have 'erogenous zones' that help us feel relaxed or sexually excited when you touch them. It's a beautiful part of having a body."

TAKEAWAYS

- Our daughters need and deserve accurate education about all parts of their sexual anatomy.
- Look at anatomical diagrams together and review with a sense of appreciation and wonder—they pick up our tone in these conversations.
- Knowing their bodies this well minimizes body shame and supports loving self-acceptance.
- Let your daughter know that the clitoris is an organ whose sole purpose is pleasure (if your child is intersex or a trans girl, make the correlation to their individual anatomy and sensory organs).
- Masturbation is completely healthy for young people.
- Reassuring our daughters that masturbation is natural helps them discover their preferences and feel more confident sexually (in the future).
- Clean hands and privacy are all that is needed.

CHAPTER TWELVE

Challenging Expectations from Porn and Social Media

When I facilitate the conversation about porn with parents, I like to share the story of a father named Adam Savage (of *Mythbusters* fame), who performed his story "Talking to My Kids about Sex in the Internet Age" at *The Moth*. He tells of learning his teen twin boys had been searching the internet for terms like "nudies" and "big boobs." He jokes in his performance, "I have my child's first porn search terms; it's almost better than their first steps!"

He then approaches his sons and tells them nervously, "The thing you gotta understand, bud, is: The internet hates women . . . Let me put it this way, if you could look into the internet like you look into someone's mind, and the internet was a dude, that dude has a problem with women."

How did we get here, and what can we do now?

Practical Guidelines

Things have changed. If we have kids near or beyond puberty age, we likely grew up having never imagined a day when access to pornography would be so widespread. Remember that the average age of first exposure to online pornography in the United States is currently seven, and six worldwide. More concerning is that 88 percent of these images are categorized as "aggressive"—either emotionally or physically violent.

In a 2009 TED Talk, advertising executive and MakeLoveNotPorn founder Cindy Gallop observed, "There is an entire generation growing up that believes that what you see in hardcore pornography is the way that you have sex. . . . My concern is especially with the young woman who . . . thinks she has to let her boyfriend [do this behavior] and pretend she likes it."

And it's not just porn teaching our kids unrealistic and harmful lessons about sex. Mainstream movies and television shows are still very male-centric in how they depict pleasure. Most still portray heterosexual sex as being defined by penile-vaginal penetration, ignoring the existence of the clitoris altogether. Too many girls and women grow up thinking something's wrong with them if they don't orgasm from penetrative sex, even though studies show only around 20 percent of women orgasm from penetration alone, without external clitoral stimulation.

For over 80 percent of women, stimulation beyond simple vaginal penetration is needed to reach orgasm. (This also means that men need not feel inadequate if thrusting alone does not satisfy their sexual partner.) "Emotional connection to a partner" also ranks very high for women in experiencing satisfying orgasms. This means that selecting sexual partners with emotional intelligence is vital. For most women, the majority of nerve endings and pleasure sensation are in the vulva (including the labia, clitoris, and vaginal opening) and the first 2–3 inches of the vaginal canal.

OPEN A DIALOGUE

First, remind your kids that porn is entertainment, and those are actors following a script. Here are some helpful, contrasting messages about healthy sex:

- Tell them that real sex is much more human.
- It can be awkward.
- People fumble.
- Bodies have hair and sweat and make sounds.
- People ask questions like, "Do you like that?"
- They stop and say, "I'm not ready for that."
- They suggest, "Here, let's try this instead."
- They check in with each other, responding to any shift in tension, and ask, "Are you okay?/Is that okay?"
- They might be playful and laugh together along the way.

We often re-create in private what we see in public. Of course, everyone can enjoy unique intimacy and authentic closeness in private—and then re-create the larger world more beautifully as a result. So, let kids know it is okay to be aroused or excited by seeing something sexual in a movie or online—the point isn't to condemn eroticism or sexual arousal. The point is to help them distinguish fantasy from reality.

Porn Addiction

Porn addiction, while presumably more common in boys, can also happen to girls. According to PornHub, about 26 percent of their 64 million users are female.

When a child (or adult) sees sexually stimulating imagery, the brain releases **dopamine**, the feel-good neurotransmitter. The spike naturally creates a reward-seeking loop, inspiring someone to return to the source of the sensation. **Oxytocin**, the love and bonding hormone, regulates dopamine levels in the body—and its levels are highest when we are physically with those we love and trust. So, when someone is alone, their oxytocin levels remain lower, allowing dopamine levels to rise and rise.

Eventually, dopamine receptors get worn out and require higher levels to achieve the same effect. This dramatic hormonal fluctuation cycle can also lead to depression and other mental health challenges.

What can a parent do?

1. Have an honest conversation with your child about the existence of online porn.

2. Install parental controls on electronic devices (see the Resources section [page 138]).

3. Check in often and offer age-appropriate outlets for stress relief.

4. Be conscious of when/how to allow social media for your child.

Social Media

New findings published in the *Wall Street Journal* in September 2021 revealed that researchers inside Instagram (owned by Meta) confirmed "32% of teen girls said that, when they feel bad about their bodies, Instagram made them feel worse."

One mother described the presence of social media and digital apps in her daughter's life as "trying to hold her back from a tornado, when all her friends are encouraging her to jump into the maelstrom." Most of us can probably relate. I have met parents who are paying their teens and tweens to stay off social media until they are 18 years old. While this may not be feasible in your family, there are simple steps we can take:

1. Choose an age limit for use and reference the Children's Online Privacy Protection Act, which bars children under 13 from

using the sites. (Kids will find ways around this—so just let them know the law is backing you up on this one.)

2. Offer only one social account at a time and set a time limit—go gradually on access.

3. Teach her to monitor her feed—being cautious of following any diet and/or exercise influencers, because the algorithms will direct this imagery to their accounts.

4. Keep all devices out of the bedroom overnight and provide a non-phone alarm clock.

5. Set aside clear off-screen times each day to connect as a family. You may meet resistance, but consistency will help ease the tension.

Like porn, the dopamine effect in everyday electronic usage can create a phenomenon where real life becomes less interesting. Try to help your child keep a balance of online time with equal amounts of offline time. This will allow her system to regulate and support a healthier relationship with the tools of technology.

Sexting

"Sexting" is the casual term for digitally sharing provocative and/or naked photos of oneself with a romantic interest. It's a pressure many girls may face, either from a love interest directly or from the numerous images they encounter of women with pursed lips and suggestive postures in media all over the internet. It's important for girls to know that images sent over phones or the internet can ultimately be seen by anyone. Kids under the age of 15 or so may not grasp just how vast and even permanent the internet can be. I encourage you to remind your daughter that any picture of herself that she sends electronically is no longer private. She has the right to be discerning about what she sends and to whom. If she's not comfortable having other people see a certain picture someday, it's best not to send it at all. Many girls have these digital tools from a young age without a lot of context on what adult life will ask of them (future employers looking them up online, etc.). Help her resist any pressure—even preemptively—to send these pictures, and give encouragement to always make choices that protect her privacy.

TAKEAWAYS

- Pornography has become the "sexual miseducation" of today, so we need to actively reeducate.
- Our daughters need to be aware of its existence from a surprisingly early age (before second grade or by age eight is best).
- Our most important job is to offer "reality checks" to help them distinguish fantasy from reality.
- Remind them again that they have the right to feel safe and enjoy any sexual experience they may have in the future.
- Having these conversations can also help prevent porn addiction (which can affect all genders).
- Map out a plan for helping your daughter balance social media use in a healthy way throughout her teen years now. Be ready to hold firm on limits and support human connection offline.

CHAPTER THIRTEEN

Promoting Healthy Relationships

Lenore and her wife, Annie, were concerned to learn about the emotional manipulation their 11-year-old daughter, Isobel, was facing via a female friend at school. They heard stories of competition, put-downs, and then sweet invitations to connect. It was baffling to their daughter, and the mothers were furious. Soon, an insight surfaced. "Our daughter told us one day that her friend started advancing on Isobel's male 'crush' and declared with delight, 'Oh, we're just like [these two characters in a teen show], how we compete over the same guy!'"

Even though the mothers were careful about the media their child saw, its influence on relationships entered Isobel's world through her friendship. So, they created a plan together. Annie had a conversation with Isobel about the value of consistency and respect in our friendships. She offered a few memories of untrustworthy friends in elementary school and how those played out in her life. Lenore agreed to periodically ask Isobel about more positive, healthier friendships and to encourage time with these friends at their home.

Our girls need to know that "drama" is not normal—it is the avoidance of confronting the true issues at hand in a healthy way. While it might sell on the ratings, it doesn't give our kids a model for how to relate to each other well.

Returning to the World Health Organization definition of sexual health, we find the phrase "free of coercion, discrimination or violence." Before relationships evolve to the point of sexual contact, healthy or unhealthy dynamics are formed. The teen years open up social choices to our girls, and new lessons are learned daily. How can we teach them to make healthy choices?

Practical Guidelines

Take the opportunity now to come up with a values statement to help steer your daughter toward high-quality friendships (for younger girls) and eventually romantic relationships (for older teens). Then, use it in casual conversation often during the adolescent years.

In our home, we say a great friendship is one where you feel free to be yourself and inspired to become even better. This is just one example of a criteria test you can offer your daughter. Another might be: "A good friend is someone who has your back when things are hard and laughs with you when things are good." Even better, come up with one together! If we're lucky, she'll hear the old saying when she's forging a new connection and use it to assess its value.

Psychologist David Richo's Five A's can be a sound guide to determine whether a relationship is forging a quality connection for both parties:

Attention—they give a healthy amount of time to the connection (neither avoidant nor smothering)

Acceptance—they show respect for who their partner truly is and affirm that in words and actions

Appreciation—they are vulnerable enough to express gratitude and say what they value in their friend/partner

Affection—they demonstrate love physically within everyone's comfort zone (which may or may not involve sex)

Allowing—they give freedom to come and go, to enjoy other pursuits and friendships

Remind your daughter that having a wide range of different friendships is valuable in itself. Our girls learn who they are through the various ways they connect and relate to others. No one person meets all of our social needs, and girls this age may need encouragement to branch out.

OPEN A DIALOGUE

Sometimes, to great parental frustration, our kids will form relationships with peers whom we don't trust or approve of. When our daughters are younger (9 to 12 or so), they may be receptive to our feedback. As adolescence approaches (13+), they are more likely to resist our interference. Yet, we need to address what we see if it concerns us.

At these times, it is best to focus on *the dynamic* instead of the kid themselves. If you find yourself dealing with a problem friend or romantic interest of your daughter's, consider this statement:

"I feel uncomfortable when I see how full of self-doubt you are after hanging out with Sammy. I'd love to see you invest your friend time and energy into someone who really lifts you up . . . But I know these are your choices to make."

Key Components:

- Speak primarily about ourselves, using the "I statement."
- Focus on your observations of the impact the connection has on your daughter.
- Express your hopes for what you'd like her to experience.
- Affirm her freedom to choose her friends.

When Relationships Are Cause for Concern

Of course, on the other end of the spectrum are the warning signs of a truly abusive relationship. According to LoveIsRespect.org, one in three adolescents in the United States experiences physical, sexual, emotional, or verbal abuse from a dating partner. So, the risk is very real among tweens and teens. We need to pay close attention.

Here are the behaviors that signal a red flag:

- pressures her into activities she may not want to do
- uses put-downs (overt or covert) and/or name-calling
- attempts to control or interfere in her relationships with others
- blames their bad behavior on her or on hard things from their past
- disregards her boundaries or guilt-trips her for setting them
- tries to isolate her from her friends and family
- threatens to expose personal secrets (or "out" them to friends or family if they are LGBTQ+) or end the relationship as a means of control
- shows extreme jealousy or accuses her of cheating without cause
- criticizes her for expressing hurt feelings and/or counter-attacks to keep themselves comfortable and unchallenged

Some ways a girl might experience abusive behaviors:

- feeling embarrassed about the abuse going on
- questioning whether it is "just them" or the actions are a big deal
- worrying their friend/partner will try to turn the community against them if they do something their partner disagrees with or if they decide to end the relationship

- managing attempts to make them feel ashamed about their sexual orientation, gender identity or expression, or sexuality in general for all orientations
- falsely concluding that their partner is the only person who will ever love them (with a special risk for LGBTQ+ kids)
- worrying that they won't be able to get help or may suffer consequences if they try to change things

When Relationships End

Many kids today (and some adults) are using the digital age as a way to hide from the hard emotional work of ending a relationship. "Ghosting," or ending a relationship without explanation by withdrawing all communication, is also a real concern. Using an email or social media post to end a relationship is never acceptable—unless someone fears for their physical safety. The one who avoids the conversation experiences lingering shame and fear, while the one left in the dark experiences uncertainty and anger.

Articulating a "no" is also crucial boundaries work. So, these are important skills for everyone involved, whether giving or receiving the news. Keep in mind, this courage applies to all aspects of her life, personal and professional.

- Teach your daughter to have the relationship-change conversation in person and in private—so everyone can move forward in the best possible way.
- Coach her in sharing specific reasons for her decision while expressing gratitude for the connection that was shared.
- Tell her how to be clear about her expectations from there: "We could get together in a month or so, just to connect," or "I'd like a few weeks of space, and then I hope we can be friends," etc.

TAKEAWAYS

- Come up with a phrase about what great friendships look like based on your family's values—and share this regularly with your daughter.
- Encourage her to have a wide range of friendships—this supports self-discovery and bolsters her when/if any relationships end.
- Watch for power imbalances and speak up when things feel off.
- Teach her the signs of healthy vs. unhealthy relationships.
- Set a family standard that relationship endings (romantic connections, for later years) are always done in person—to guide her in giving and receiving interpersonal respect.
- Normalize having difficult conversations because it supports her confidence in all aspects of life.

CHAPTER FOURTEEN

Exploring Safer Sex

Do you remember the old "running the bases" metaphor for sex? Going to first base, second base . . . home run? Well, sexuality educator Al Vernacchio has offered us a new metaphor, one that encourages both mutual pleasure and safety: pizza.

In his TED Talk, "Sex Needs a New Metaphor," Vernacchio notes how "when we get together with someone for pizza, we're not competing with them, we're looking for an experience that we will share that's satisfying for both of us." Poignantly, as it relates to safer sex, he also concludes, ". . . and what's the first thing you do? You talk about it . . . what you want. You talk about what you like. You might even negotiate, 'How do you feel about pepperoni?' . . . isn't it all about, 'What's our pleasure?'"

As you'll see in this chapter, safer sex for our kids is rooted in the idea that 1) sex is a mutually enjoyable activity, and 2) to have that safe, enjoyable experience, you need to first talk about it . . .

Practical Guidelines

One of the greatest benefits of starting conversations with our daughters about sex is that it increases the likelihood she'll talk to future partners about sex before it happens—which is crucial to enjoying safer sex. So, let's start preparing to have specific conversations about STIs and contraceptive information.

Sexually Transmitted Infections (STIs)

At 8 to 10 years old, your daughter can safely learn about the existence of STIs—sexually transmitted infections (updated from years ago, when they were referred to as sexually transmitted diseases, or STDs). If your daughter is 11 to 14, she needs to know that there are bacterial STIs—which can be treated with medication—and viral STIs that stay with you your whole life. If she is 15 or older, it is time to give her details about each STI so she can be aware of symptoms and courses for prevention. Girls develop at different rates, so this timeline should be adjusted based on your daughter's unique development, especially if you think she may be sexually active earlier.

While it's not easy to imagine our children encountering any of the infections outlined in chapter 3 (page 30), it can be a reminder of the importance and power of prevention. Letting them know how normal it is to get tested before *every sexual encounter with a new partner*—whether penetrative or not—can literally be lifesaving. This means they have to talk about protection before any contact with their new partner. Planned Parenthood clinics often have free or low-cost testing available to people of all ages. Many also have free condoms available, with no questions asked.

Once kids understand how easy and simple the tests are, intimidation also decreases. A simple blood, urine, and/or saliva test is usually enough to rule out the most common infections. An exam may not even be required.

Safety from Unwanted Pregnancy

It is helpful for everyone to understand how conception and pregnancy occur. You can safely share this information with your daughter at age 10 or 11. Your child can learn both when she is fertile and the role of semen (the fluid that someone with a penis and testes ejaculates) in pregnancy (see Resources, page 138). While it is rare, pregnancies have occurred even without intercourse, when semen is near the opening of the vagina.

Discuss birth control options with your daughter before she enters high school—even if you don't expect her to become sexually active in those years. Just hearing you talk about **condoms, the pill, IUDs** (and other contraception mentioned in chapter 3 [page 30]) will take a lot of the mystique out of the process. Whenever parents can reduce intimidation, we are empowering our kids.

It's also important to let them know that even if they are on birth control such as the pill or have an IUD, they need to advocate for themselves and require sexual partners with penises to wear condoms to protect from STIs. Everyone needs to know about using dental dams (latex protective barriers for safe oral sex) as well. Just be sure to check for a latex allergy in advance.

Am I Encouraging My Daughter to Become Sexually Active?

It's natural to worry that sharing these details will somehow give a message of permission or encouragement to our girls to be sexually active. For now, be reassured that research has shown us otherwise. More detailed information will make your child less vulnerable to unhealthy risk-taking—and it may help steer her away from potentially unwanted experiences.

For example, I've heard plenty of stories from families about abstinence messages yielding unintended consequences. When a girl has taken an abstinence pledge, she often then hears from peers that anal and/or oral sex "do not count." In these cases, a girl is often less prepared to prevent STIs—or to make a decision that supports her well-being. While abstinence can definitely be recommended as part of sexual health, please take the extra step to communicate the various ways young people are sexually active. Help distinguish her options for pleasurable contact she *can* currently enjoy. There are options for mutual pleasure—like kissing, holding hands, and mutual masturbation—that someone refraining from vaginal intercourse can enjoy with much lower risk of STIs.

OPEN A DIALOGUE

If your daughter has a love interest from age 12 or older, you can confidently introduce the topic of STI protection and birth control, even if it feels way too early. She may groan in response, but she'll likely be immensely relieved for the honest check-in.

"Do you and your sweetie have a plan for birth control if you ever get to that point?"

"What have you and your girlfriend/boyfriend/partner talked about for STI protection?"

"Would you know how to get birth control if you needed it?"

"What do you know about STIs?"

"You know, I am happy to get you the protection you need, just in case."

Try sprinkling the topic throughout a few weeks, instead of mounting anxieties for one big talk. The opener, "Have you thought about this?" can be followed up with, "So, what have you decided for STI protection?" a week later. Keep the topic neutral and supportive, and she will trust that you have her back.

TAKEAWAYS

- Tell your daughter that people always have the conversation about STIs (and birth control, where relevant) before sexual activity.
- Let her know how simple the process is—and let her know you are available to help.
- Inform her of the difference between bacterial STIs (can be treated) vs. viral STIs (stay with you your whole life).
- Talk about birth control options with your daughter before she enters high school.
- Visit the Planned Parenthood website to review birth control options, even much earlier than needed.
- Discuss what sexual activities are acceptable at what ages (especially if abstinence is part of your message).
- Remind her that safety is always her right, no matter who she is with or what anyone is doing.

CHAPTER FIFTEEN

Encouraging Girls to Communicate Wants, Needs, and Limits

Robert, a 34-year-old single dad, tells of taking his eight-year-old daughter, Camille, to a buffet-style restaurant during a long road trip. She excitedly filled her plate with veggies and meat and slid down to the dessert section to find the vanilla pudding essentially empty. She looked to Robert to express her dismay. He said, "Well, you just need to ask someone to refill it."

Just then, an elderly woman with a restaurant apron walked nearby. Robert motioned that she would be someone to ask. Camille approached the employee confidently and said, "Excuse me, but the vanilla pudding is empty and needs to be refilled." The woman responded gruffly, "Well, you're an outspoken little lady, aren't you?" Robert locked eyes with the woman and exclaimed joyfully, "Yes, that's right, and I am very proud of her."

For Camille, that was all that mattered.

Practical Guidelines

The early years are a chance to give girls the message, in so many ways, that her needs and experience matter. As girls leave the "nest" of the home and venture into the social world of peers—and soon employment and academic achievement—their relationship to their inner knowing can falter. Combine an innate developmental task with a culture that provides near-constant electronic stimulation—and a girl can lose herself and her way.

As parents, we can help create an environment that supports our daughter's self-awareness. Certain sports and outdoor recreational activities may naturally create this space. Yet, being among your friends can also distract you from tuning into your deeper truth. This is a loud world, and sometimes a girl needs intentional quiet to hear herself.

Try these simple tools to help a girl discover her wants, needs, and limits:

- schedule some offline downtime for your daughter a few days each week—or each day, if possible
- encourage journaling or drawing as quiet reflection activities—research published in *Anxiety, Stress & Coping* has shown that, in a 12-week trial, 20 minutes of expressive journaling each day significantly lowered depressive and anxious symptoms within one month, and increased overall resilience by two months
- help her to move her body in silence if she is the more active type—such as yoga, stretching, running, swimming, or other forms of individual exercise
- begin teaching her about mindfulness exercises such as deep breathing and guided and silent meditation

Help Your Daughter Approach the World to Meet Her Needs

Even a child of eight or nine can be encouraged to handle her own monetary exchange at a business with a friendly employee. If you are buying something for your child, ask her to greet the cashier, hear the payment request, and handle the money.

Let your six-year-old be the one to place her order at the ice cream shop. Does your 11-year-old want a certain book from the library? Help her be the one to make the call and ask if it's on the shelves. Is your 14-year-old interested in team sports? Have her be the one to reach out to the coach to ask about openings.

Of course, these examples will vary dramatically depending on your family's unique circumstances and life experience. What opportunities could you find where you could encourage your daughter to be proactive and assertive about meeting her needs? This will help her grow her autonomy and resourcefulness. When you see her advocating for herself, it's important to reflect back to her that, yes, she does have the right to respectfully ask for what she needs—regardless of how well her requests are received by the world around her.

Finally, it's also important to note that a girl's voice need not be loud to be effective. Naturally shy or introverted girls are just as capable of speaking their needs and limits as more extroverted ones. When it comes to speaking up for oneself, it's not about volume, but the power and clarity in the truths spoken.

Limits as the Edge of Needs

Part of advocating for our needs is being able to express a limit. When our daughter needs rest, the limit is "I can't go to the party tonight." When she needs to tend her own assignments, it looks like, "No, I need to go through my list first before helping you." Limit setting can be a gracious and honest practice for people of all ages. We can remind our daughters, simply, that letting others down in small ways is a natural part of being true to ourselves.

For a six-year-old, boundaries can mean learning how to say, "This is my room. I don't want you to come in here." For an eight-year-old, it might be, "That's my favorite shirt. You can't borrow it." A tween could learn, "That's personal," in choosing to not share information. Each age and skillset builds upon the previous, to navigate boundaries within greater intimacy down the line. For more on Boundaries, please see chapter 7 (page 61).

OPEN A DIALOGUE

Assertiveness is rarely recognized for the powerful, healthy stance that it is. Asking for what we want (and being clear about what we don't want) is kind because it allows for directness, clarity, and more harmonious relationships. Let's clear up some of the differences between assertive communication and what can become aggressive or irresponsible.

Irresponsible: "Gee, those dumplings smell really good, and I'm so hungry . . ."

Assertive: "May I have one of your dumplings?"

Aggressive: "Some people never offer to share, even when they have too much!"

In the teen dating years, this becomes . . .

Irresponsible: "Sure, I'd love to go to the party with you"—then avoiding all contact when the person follows up.

Assertive: "Thanks, but I'm not sure of my plans yet, and I need to think it over."

Aggressive: "Like I'd go to a party with you," (tone of disgust)—then going with their good friend instead.

- Start now by giving a message that asking for what you want and need is the kindest thing to do in any inter-personal situation.
- Let her know that letting others down by being honest is a sign of great strength.
- Make sure she has time to tune in to herself, offline, and in personal reflection—especially as her social life picks up in the later teen years.
- Teach your daughter about money—and have her ask for what she wants in stores, etc.
- Take excellent care of yourself by addressing any grief or uneasiness as you watch your daughter rise as a confident, assertive woman.

CHAPTER SIXTEEN

Instilling a Comprehensive Understanding of Consent

"Consent" has become a hot-topic word, especially since the rise of the #MeToo movement in 2017. Many of these "hot topics" can feel delicate or volatile to meet directly (and well) as parents.

Knowing how consent is achieved, understanding where/when consent is not possible, and seeing how these concepts apply to sex as well as regular life empowers girls to move with greater confidence. As with many earlier lessons about bodies and relationships, this is a great opportunity for you to help your daughter apply these principles to her own sexuality.

Let's start by breaking down the concept of *consent* into manageable pieces.

Practical Guidelines

Consent is always the responsibility of both people involved. So, whether our girls are requesting closeness or responding to a request, clear communication skills are needed on both sides.

In so many ways, we can teach our daughters to be forthright in giving a clear "yes," "no," or "I don't know." According to research, girls more often use qualifying phrases such as, "*I think* I don't want to," or "*I might* be into that." As parents, we can coach them to be clearer and more concise. "No, thanks," and "Yes, that sounds great," are alternatives. The difference may seem subtle, but it is profound in practice.

Of course, all of this builds up to dating relationships where physical closeness is navigated.

Affirmative and Enthusiastic Consent

Fortunately, conversations around sex and consent have evolved from focusing on simply the absence of a "no" to looking for affirmative and enthusiastic consent—the clear presence of a "yes!" Body language can enhance spoken language by conveying enthusiasm, but smiles and nods alone do not equate to consent. First must be the question, "Are you okay with this?" and then must be the positive answer, "Yes." We need to be talking during sex to achieve consent, and young people need to know this. Confirming mutual interest before sexual contact is an ideal start, and agreement that activity can stop at any time reinforces enthusiastic consent.

Limits to Consent and Sex

According to the law (and basic respect), in most states, a person cannot give consent to sexual activity while under the influence of drugs or alcohol. While blood alcohol limits are often unclear or undefined legally, this concept is useful in helping our daughters understand that *our decision-making deserves clarity.* There is a lot of gray area when it comes to men (most often) offering women (the common recipient) alcoholic drinks, and how that affects what she will or will not agree to.

For older teens, it's important to be aware that about *half of all sexual assaults involve alcohol,* according to the National Institute of Alcohol Abuse and Alcoholism. Some ways to help prevent such assaults include teaching a young girl to (later in life) only ever get her own drink, or watch a bartender pour for her directly, and to keep her drink with her. There are four classifications of "date rape drugs" that cause forgetfulness, loss of consciousness, weakness, and more. This includes alcohol. Learning this information can give a girl agency in navigating social situations with alcohol and drugs.

Encourage your daughter to always attend social gatherings with a close and trusted friend, and to talk with them in advance about what she does and does not want to do that night, sexually. If she is able to be clear—and to have an ally helping her stay true to her preferences—an unfortunate situation can be avoided. (See Chapter 5 [page 50] for more on the "no consequences conversation" and having her back.)

In the US, the legal "age of consent" also varies state to state, ranging from age 16 to 18. So, a child must be at least this old to give consent to sexual activity. When a larger age differential exists between partners, and one is over 18, sex can be considered statutory rape. The law exists because age difference can create a power imbalance, making consent impossible and abuse the more accurate term. Some states have a "close in age" exemption, decriminalizing sexual activity when both partners are under the age of consent.

Coercion

Remember, the definition of sexual health from the World Health Organization includes the phrase "free of coercion" (see page viii). So, what does that mean? Coercion can be physical, social, emotional, psychological, or fear- and/or shame-based. If a girl arrives at "agreement" to sex under any kind of duress, it is not enthusiastic consent. It may even be rape. Some common tactics to identify in advance include:

▸ telling her she likes something when she hasn't said so herself
▸ comparing her to her friends or peers, leveraging pressure for social acceptance
▸ plying her for sympathy and/or implying that she needs to "make him feel better" with sex
▸ using put-downs to confuse her ability to clearly set limits
▸ verbally harassing her until she agrees to sex to make it stop
▸ suggesting that "cool" or socially acceptable people always do certain sexual things
▸ threatening to expose something personal about her if she does not agree
▸ threatening to harm someone/something they care about if she doesn't comply

Simply put, coercion is what happens when someone has not accepted a "no" and continues to push for what they want. It can happen in all kinds of situations—and is intensified by the inherent vulnerability of sex. This is why early guidance in setting boundaries and limits is so crucial. Being able to tolerate someone else's disappointment and still hold firm is one benefit of earlier boundaries practice.

Lastly, make sure your daughter understands that her freedom to choose what sexual activity she engages in, with whom, and when is always non-negotiable; it's an absolute right. Being in a relationship doesn't mean she "owes" anyone sex. Agreeing to something once doesn't obligate her to ever agree again. If she is unclear on whether it is an enthusiastic "yes" for her or her partner, then it means "no" until they both know what they want.

Coercion can cause confusion, regret, and lasting trauma. Accepting someone's limits is a strong indicator of love and respect. Help your daughter practice simple expressions like, "I'm not ready for that," and "I don't want to have sex. Don't ask again." Clear and concise is the best way to respond to even subtle coercion.

OPEN A DIALOGUE

A great place to start the conversation about consent with your daughter is by watching Blue Seat Studios' popular videos about consent with her (see the Resources section [page 138]).

If your daughter is age 6 to 11, or you want to start with basics first, try the video "Consent for Kids." It introduces the concept of "bodily autonomy" and clarifies our rights around consent. It also includes subtle mention of dynamics that accompany child sexual abuse and gives notice of behaviors that signal a red flag. I'd include it in any conversation around preventing abuse, even for teens who may not have had this education elsewhere.

For girls age 12 and up, the "Tea Consent" video is a funny, direct, and honest way of talking about consent. It's lighthearted enough that your daughter is unlikely to cringe in embarrassment (since sex is only mentioned at the end). I recommend watching it with young people of any gender to enjoy a valuable discussion.

TAKEAWAYS

- Clear communication is the foundation of a solid understanding of consent: "yes," "no," "I don't know." Teach your daughter to be concise.
- Make sure she knows that consent applies to belongings, personal information, and what she does with her own body.
- Help her understand the limits of consent, and what coercion may look like. Teach her to trust and honor her gut instincts—if it doesn't feel right, it's not right.
- Celebrate the idea of "enthusiastic consent," a clear and resounding "yes!" and how to give it and recognize it in others.

CHAPTER SEVENTEEN

Affirming Gender Identity and Sexuality

As your daughter approaches puberty, you will have many opportunities to affirm her gender and her sexuality. Even if your child is cisgender (identifies with her assigned sex at birth), you will still be making choices—even unconscious ones—that affirm or negate the woman she is becoming.

Sometimes, as adults, we forget just how harrowing the process of identity formation can be. Rarely is it ever a straight line of becoming—expect lots of turns and detours along the way. Reflect back for a moment on your own sexual maturity . . . Were there messages you received that denied or canceled your gender identity? Were you told that "Nice girls don't do that," or "Don't be a sissy," or "That's not a ladylike thing to do," or "Man up"? Each of these statements negate an inherent part of a young person's being. It is social messaging that unintentionally stifles growth and self-expression.

Even more poignantly, were there messages that denied, suppressed, or shamed your natural sexuality? Because you are here now, we have an opportunity to give something more supportive to our own daughters.

In this chapter, we'll explore ways to create and deliver messaging that will affirm your daughter's identity and sexuality. Remember, a primary developmental task of adolescence is integrating sexuality into one's identity. It's a universal milestone for growth. This task will mark successful progression in her full growth as a dynamic and self-assured woman. Here we go.

Practical Guidelines

In chapter 3, we covered the basics of gender and sexual identity. Here we will explore more ways you can support your child as they discover and assert these aspects of their identity.

Supporting Your Daughter's Gender Identity and Expression

As a reminder, gender identity is a concept in the mind, someone's understanding of who they are inside—an understanding that often starts very young. Gender expression includes the range of personal choices—clothing, hair, vocal expressions, and pronouns—that reflect who they are inside. A girl can choose non-traditionally female gender expressions (such as shorter hair or traditionally masculine clothing, etc.) and still identify as a woman.

The American Psychiatric Association makes an important distinction in supporting gender-diverse people: "Gender Affirming Therapy is a therapeutic stance that focuses on affirming a patient's gender identity and does not try to 'repair' it." This clarifies that gender is not something to be fixed; rather, it is an inner reality simply needing outer confirmation. It's about affirming who a child already knows themselves to be.

Remember, even though the terminology and awareness are new, these are not novel experiences. People have always lived a range of identities, expressions, and orientations. It is only recently that we have the benefit of a better way to talk about it.

Generally, a young person wants their outer expression to match their inner understanding of who they are. Some teens will experiment with a range of expressions throughout puberty, and this is healthy and normal, too. Sometimes, our kids will need help to affirm their gender, so they can live with a sense of peace and rightness.

PUBERTY FOR THE GENDER DIVERSE

If your child is transgender or questioning their gender identity, the changes of puberty can be especially alarming and may lead to gender dysphoria—the feeling of distress that arises from a mismatch of identity and anatomy. This sense of unease may be so intense that it leads to depression, anxiety, and even suicide. If your child is experiencing gender dysphoria, you may want to consider supporting them with puberty blockers. These are medicines that pause puberty while a young person decides which steps to take to live their healthiest life. They block the influx of estrogen or testosterone that lead to periods, breast growth, and/or the deepening of the voice and growth of facial/body hair. They are entirely reversible, and buy valuable time and relief. Find a supportive doctor and schedule an initial consultation. Please see the Resources section (page 138) for more information.

Supporting Your Daughter's Sexual Orientation

It is valuable to always speak to your daughter about sexuality with the added disclaimer "no matter whom you end up being attracted to." This doesn't encourage a different orientation (as sexual orientation is innate and not subject to suggestion). You actually wind up creating necessary safety for her and for any friends who may be LGBTQ+. If your daughter is attracted to the same gender or all genders, you'll be a primary source of acceptance and affirmation for who she truly is.

"Coming out" is the process of disclosure about sexual orientation to someone in your life. Heterosexual people generally don't need to go through the experience (as opposite-gender attraction is usually assumed in our society). For girls who are lesbian, bisexual, or pansexual, revealing this truth to a parent, friend, teacher, or extended family member can be nerve-racking. The very best response is to express joy for her self-discovery. For a girl who is gay, lesbian, bi, or pan, learning to "come out" to all kinds of people is its own self-development exercise. Teach her to gauge levels of acceptance and safety in others and reveal accordingly. Most of all, be ready to be that secure base of acceptance as she continually brings who she truly is to more and more people in her life.

Coming out is different for trans children. For trans girls (girls who were assigned male at birth) who may not be publicly out, early dating in the teen years can be especially challenging. The real human needs for emotional connection and personal safety are heightened during this time. She will need extra courage from those around her to make it a strong and successful beginning. We still live in a society where trans teens often have to fight for their identity and their rights. So, peer support—in addition to your unconditional acceptance—can make a huge difference. PFLAG is a great place to start for resources, connections, and support. (See Resources, page 138.)

OPEN A DIALOGUE

Because gender and sexuality are such sensitive topics, it helps to stay aware of language that is shaming versus affirming. Here are some helpful examples of shaming statements and ways to adjust your own language:

- Instead of "You're not the kind of girl who dresses like that," try using a "what" or "how" question to invite retrospection, being mindful of tone: "What is it about that outfit you like the most?" or "How do you feel when you put on those clothes?"

- Instead of "Don't you think that's kind of butch?" consider a neutral statement of awe over how things change: "Wow, it's exciting for me to see how much more accepting your generation is with self-expression."

- Instead of saying "No one else's daughter is dating this young!" offer an expression of your concerns, followed by trust: "I just get scared that you will face negative consequences for being so romantically involved. But this is a new time, and I'll trust you to discover what works best for you."

- For moments that clearly cross the line, say: "I can't let you make that choice because I'm concerned for your safety. In a few years, if this still feels like the right choice, I will step back and let you try it then." (Make it about maturity level and not who she is becoming.)

TAKEAWAYS

- Gender is affirmed by choices like hair, clothing, mannerisms, pronouns, name choices, and sometimes by medical support.
- Gender identity is a concept in the mind—separate from expression or sexual attraction (orientation).
- Puberty blockers are one way to pause the changes of sexual maturity for a gender-diverse child—and they're reversible.
- Offer supportive messaging about gender identity and sexuality starting when your child is young. Be especially conscious of how you speak about LGBTQ+ people in the media or in your community.
- Even when we struggle, we can always find a supportive message.
- Take some time to craft a handful of universally accepting messages about sexuality and gender now; they'll come in handy many times along the way.

PART IV

FREQUENTLY ASKED QUESTIONS, ANSWERED

Some of the richest moments in my career have been facilitating parent nights or seminars with parents who want to support their kids in healthy sexuality. A range of values, cultures, and religions would naturally reveal themselves—and I always regarded the courage it takes to bring these questions to a group. For this section, I hope you will see yourself reflected in at least a few of these situations, which represent some of the most common questions I have received as a sex educator. We are more alike than different when it comes to caring about our kids and sexuality.

1. How do I get my daughter to wait to have sex?

I encourage you to frame this as a series of criteria a relationship must pass through to become worthy of that closeness.

It's okay to set a minimum time frame (six months, one year, etc.) that a couple needs to grow together. If your values involve not having sex until marriage, be sure to offer your daughter alternatives for what activity is acceptable before marriage.

Have a series of "Have they earned your trust?" questions for assessing whether that relationship is ready for the vulnerability and responsibility of sex, including making a plan for contraception, where appropriate. Revisit the STI conversation (see chapter 14 [page 104]) and remind her that being able to have these talks is crucial before a couple is ready for sex.

2. I don't want to teach my eight-year-old about sex yet because I want her to enjoy her innocence as long as possible. Do I really need to give her all this information so young?

These are personal choices, and there is no universal right answer. I respect how proactive information can seem contrary to childhood. Many of us had childhoods that were blissfully unaware and want the same for our daughters. But it is simply a different world today. Information is so accessible now that being uninformed can be scarier—and more dangerous—for kids than being aware of what she might see in advance. It can also lead to a girl being ill-equipped to deal with the very real threat of sexual exploitation.

Most of my clients who endured some kind of child sexual abuse or teen pregnancy were excessively sheltered. It can feel counterintuitive, but the child who is astute and aware is far less likely to be sexually abused. A girl who has encouragement to talk—and a parent to talk to—is less likely to suffer in silence if she encounters abuse. She is also less likely to make reckless choices about sex later in life.

3. My 10-year-old is more physically developed than most of her peers and is being bullied at school. The sexual undertone of the comments really worries me. How can I support her?

At this age, it's totally appropriate to have meetings with her teachers and/or administrators about your concerns. A few things to make clear:

1. What is their policy on discipline for harassment? Are there procedures for reporting and consequences for students who violate standards?

2. Use the phrase "sexual harassment," even if it feels extreme. There are federal protections in place (Title IX for education), and going in with significant language will help employees take this seriously.

3. Decide whether to involve the parent/s of kids who are behaving poorly. It may be the right choice. Your daughter may have resistance to this, for fear of embarrassment. But overall, addressing it thoroughly and quickly is best.

4. Lastly, empower her with a few tools to respond to sexual teasing in the moment. A simple command, such as "Don't talk to me like that," may be best. Sometimes, the power of "getting a kid upset" underlies the draw of bullying. Anger is appropriate, yet a composed message may help minimize the attention.

Hopefully this becomes a powerful lesson in standing up for herself that steers her toward better environments over and over again.

4. I caught my daughter experimenting sexually with another child—she's only 11. Do I need to talk to that child's parents, or can I make this a lesson for our family?

When these things happen, the first question must be whether everyone involved agreed and felt safe. Even an age difference of one year can create a power imbalance that prevents some kids from speaking up. So, start by asking your child these questions.

As for the parents, the answer lies in the golden rule—and in your goals for a supportive network in parenting. Ask yourself, "If the tables were turned, would I want to be informed?" Of course, family needs and values will vary. But other parents can be powerful allies in raising our kids well.

Also consider the role of secrecy in perpetuating shame. The kids may be embarrassed, but breaking the silence can bring things into the light and break the spell. If you decide to talk to the parents, I encourage you to open with your desire to help both kids feel safe and comfortable with sexuality.

5. What do you think about middle schoolers having co-ed sleepovers? My child says all the families are okay with it, but I'm not so sure.

Remember, tweens and teens may have a skewed perception about what "everyone" is doing. First, distinguish between one-on-one mixed-gender sleepovers and group sleepovers. Is it a longtime opposite-sex friend still wanting extended connection? Is it a group of kids of different genders all sleeping together in one family's basement/play area?

As parents, we can be very clear about our expectations for boundaries with contact with other kids overnight. I'd say, first, reach out to the parent hosting and ask what the arrangement is. Second, lay down your expectations, whether that's staying in separate rooms or beds all night or more directly not engaging in sexual activity yet. This is a great opportunity to talk with your daughter about her sexual choices.

Also remember that sexual orientation varies, and guide the conversation for all possible situations.

6. My daughter, age 13, came out to me as lesbian earlier this year. I'm happy for her, and she seems confident in her orientation. How do I support sexual health for a girl who loves girls when I don't understand it myself?

First, congratulations on raising a child who is confident and open with you about her sexuality. A few points to keep in mind:

▶ Make sure she understands the importance of STI prevention and the options available to her. Even with a reduced risk of pregnancy, she still needs sexual health care.
▶ Help her make regular appointments for a Pap smear and STI screening as soon as she is sexually active—bisexual and lesbian women tend to have a higher risk for infections and less treatment.
▶ Remember to consider the HPV (human papilloma virus) vaccine and PrEP.
▶ Start now looking for LGBTQ+ friendly and supportive health care providers. This will help her continue her care as she becomes more independent.
▶ Help her stay connected to other LGBTQ+ young people.
▶ Consider joining an organization like PFLAG (formerly known as Parents, Families, and Friends of Lesbians and Gays).

7. What about cutting? I've heard this is a problem among teen girls.

Cutting and other forms of self-harm tend to indicate she is dealing with immense stress—often social isolation and feelings of helplessness. Similar to some disordered eating, it arises as a momentary "stress-relief" strategy, a coping mechanism that brings a temporary feeling of control. Cutting usually does not indicate suicidal tendencies, but the behavior is clearly an alarm and a cry for help.

First, take the behavior seriously. The child is overwhelmed, isolated, and needing support. Nervous tension can manifest in the body, so redirecting them to physically strenuous activities or artistic expression can help.

Most importantly, social support is a great reliever of stress. If you can, help her connect with supportive peers. If the behavior continues, seek a counselor or trusted support person that can help her learn how to manage her big feelings.

8. My daughter has a developmental disability, and I have a whole host of worries about her and sex. Can she expect to enjoy this in a healthy way when she is older?

The main issue around sex that affects kids with developmental disabilities and neurodiversity (such as cerebral palsy, autism spectrum disorder, central auditory processing disorder, attention deficit disorder, and Down syndrome) is insecurity and self-consciousness. Most people without physical disabilities also struggle with shame or doubts about their bodies—which is only aggravated by awareness of being physically or cognitively "different."

Beginning with an understanding of "how normal different is" can help minimize any self-doubt. Seek out media that offers positive, diverse representations of relationships.

The other crucial piece is to teach her to seek a balanced relationship of equal power. This is absolutely possible. It may or may not mean choosing a partner with disabilities; true compassion can arise in any body. But, help her choose relationships where she can feel herself to be on equal footing.

9. My daughter's friend has an older sister who recently had an abortion. She mentioned this to me, and I kind of froze. I do want to go back and bring it up again, but it's such a heated topic! What can I say?

This is a great opportunity to teach your daughter about sex and your family's values. So many consequences can seem "hypothetical" to the adolescent mind.

There are a few kinds of messages I would guard against: shaming a woman for becoming pregnant only creates an environment of unsafety. Two people were involved and responsible for that pregnancy. Pitying and "poor her" responses also reinforce a helplessness for women around sex. This is unlikely to be helpful.

The best angle for the conversation may be one focused on the choices available to the woman leading up to conceiving. How might she have been able to avoid pregnancy? Access to information? Birth control? Was there consent?

There is no right answer here. But, there is a child watching her parent for signs of how safe she might be if she found herself in a similar situation. Kids of all ages need to feel secure and accepted within their families. So, reopen the conversation based on life choices and your willingness to support her—and a rich dialogue will likely unfold.

10. My daughter keeps asking about my first time having sex, how old I was, what it was like, etc. This feels too personal to share! I'm worried I'm giving her a negative message by just shying away from it over and over . . .

First, you have absolutely no obligation to share personal information outside your comfort zone.

Fortunately, you can fully address these questions while protecting your privacy. For example, "How old were you?" carries a deeper curiosity—the universal "What is normal?" Most likely, she's looking for context on what people do. You can respond, "That is private to me. What is it you really need to know?"

11. My daughter is going through her first major breakup at 16, and I'm worried about how she's handling it. She just seems inaccessible and not open to my support now.

This can be so heart-wrenching for a parent. A good angle (if you haven't tried it yet) would be to just ask her to explain it to you from a place of complete unknowing. What is this like for her? Sometimes, affirming the uniqueness of her experience can help bring down walls of defense.

Grief is such a unique and individual process. Is she falling behind in school? Losing sleep? Gaining or losing weight? Unless you see signs of the grief impacting her health or responsibilities, she may just need time. Sometimes, giving real space to mourn is just what we need to move forward completely.

If she won't open up to you at all, try getting a few books on love, grieving, and trust from the library and leaving them out for her. It's a secondary gesture to help her know she's not alone. A simple, repeated message of "I'm here" may be your best option for a while.

12. I tend to think a woman should be the one to talk to girls about sex and vice versa with men. I'll talk to our son when he gets to be this age. My wife still wants me to talk to our daughter (age 12). But I'm afraid I'll just mess it up.

It is so worthwhile to challenge these assumptions about where sexual health information comes from. I'd reflect it back to you this way: What are you saying to her about sex by not broaching the topic? That men don't talk to women about sex? That it's beneath men to deal with emotional conversations?

I'm guessing at her interpretations, of course. The point is that she is likely receiving a message from your lack of communication on the topic. If your daughter is heterosexual or bisexual, and romantic relationships with men are likely part of her future, you absolutely have a lot to offer her in these conversations. It may feel incredibly awkward, but the risk is worth the long-term reward.

Try opening with a hope for her future relationships. As much as possible, frame this in the positive, or, as what you *do* want. For most parents, it's easier to call up our fears and what we want to avoid. Instead, imagine the best possible outcomes for her—and put these into language: "When you start dating, I hope you [choose someone who honors you completely/choose someone who helps you feel like you can do anything in this world/etc.]."

She is watching you for signals and learning about sex from nearly every other part of her life. Let her know you as a positive source of information and guidance on this, too.

13. My daughter just told me she was sexually assaulted at a party. What should I do?

First, thank her for telling you (especially when you are calm) and reassure her that she did nothing wrong. It was not her fault. Then, start a conversation about what she wants to do. If there was an age differential, talk together about the law and statutory rape (see chapter 16 [page 114]). Involving the police may feel big and intimidating (and even unsafe), but having a police report keeps options open for future legal action. Make a plan for her to feel safe day to day (for instance, if she sees this person at school). If she needs personal time to recenter, consider allowing a break from her usual responsibilities. Reaching out to the parent(s) of the person who did this may be another step—one to take at your daughter's agreement and pacing. Within a comfortable time frame (ideally 4 to 6 weeks), make a plan to address this behavior with someone in authority, whether police, school leaders, parents, or an attorney. What goes unaddressed could continue. As much as possible, seek her permission before acting. Lastly, make sure to offer to get her Plan B (the "morning-after pill") or access to PEP (post-exposure prophylaxis for HIV prevention) if necessary. With you as a compassionate ally, she will recover more smoothly. It may also be wise to find a therapist with whom she can work through the trauma, especially if she is showing any signs of PTSD. RAINN is an excellent resource for victims of sexual assault (see the Resources section [page 138]).

14. I'm scared that my daughter's relationship with her boyfriend isn't healthy and may even be abusive. How do I bring this up to her without pushing her away?

Start small and allow a lot of space in between conversations for your daughter to integrate your concerns with her own experience. For example, "I noticed you were so down after spending time with your boyfriend last week. Do you want to talk about it?" If you get a "no," leave it for a few days. Come back with, "I keep thinking about the kinds of relationships I hope you'll have . . . are you open to hearing my ideals for you?" Again, if you get a "no," give time and resume in a few days. Small doses of your concern may be more tolerable than a perceived "interrogation." Tell her you are there to support her, no matter what she is going through.

15. My child recently announced they are nonbinary and use the pronouns "they/them." Our extended family is very conservative, and I know they will have a problem with this. How can I best support my child while also maintaining a relationship with everyone else?

Well, you can maintain a relationship with everyone else, but you may have to accept that it will carry some tensions until everyone adjusts. Your child is your responsibility and has needs that other family members do not. The best approach will be to prepare for ways you can stand in solidarity with your child while expressing a desire to continue contact with the rest. Get ready to set limits with extended family—lay out what will and will not be tolerated when your child is around them. If these are not respected, pull back. Remind yourself often that this period of strain will show your child what they mean to you and to the larger world. Most importantly, make sure you are doing your best to support your child's identity and pronouns. Even if others aren't respecting them, knowing you've got their back will go a very long way. You may even teach your family about the value of loyalty in action.

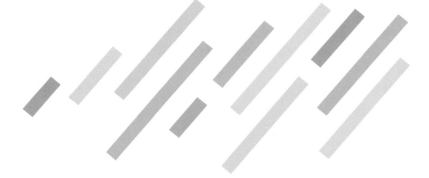

RESOURCES

This list includes books, podcasts, and videos that can either be used by parents for additional information and support—or be shared with your child. A few (with ages mentioned) are appropriate to give as gifts to your daughter. Just be sure to follow up with a conversation or two. Books for kids are great prompts for something you can reference together, and to facilitate your own conversations.

Sexual Health and Puberty

Planned Parenthood—One of the best resources about sexual health in general, and teen sexual health specifically
PlannedParenthood.org/learn/teens

Sex Ed Rescue—A wonderfully comprehensive, sex-positive resource for parents of kids of all ages, genders, orientations, and more
SexEdRescue.com

Scarleteen: Sex Ed for the Real World—Inclusive, comprehensive, supportive sexuality and relationships info for teens and emerging adults
Scarleteen.com

How to Be a Girl—A podcast about raising a young transgender girl
HowToBeAGirlPodcast.com

"Nourishing Our Young Women Forwards and Backwards: The Red Party," by Vanessa Osage—My article about menarche and puberty rites of passage.
VanessaOsage.Medium.com/nourishing-our-young-women
-forwards-and-backwards-the-red-party-f71ccaf0f7b6

Honoring Our Cycles, by Katie Singer—A great resource with simple language explaining the menstrual cycle, charting to know when a period is likely to begin, and how conception occurs

Environmental Working Group Database for Product Safety—A list of skin care products that are verified by the EWG
EWG.org/ewgverified/products.php?type=skin-care

OMGYES—A wonderful resource to help people of all genders understand the basics of women's pleasure
OMGYES.com

Mental Health

The American Academy of Child and Adolescent Psychiatry, Psychiatrist Finder Tool
AACAP.org/aacap/Families_and_Youth/Resources/CAP_Finder.aspx

"Teen Suicide: Understanding the Risk and Getting Help"
NewsInHealth.NIH.gov/2019/09/teen-suicide

Psychology Today, Find a Therapist
PsychologyToday.com/us

Dopamine Nation: Finding Balance in the Age of Indulgence, by Anna Lembke

Media

Common Sense Media—A leading source of entertainment and technology recommendations for families
CommonSenseMedia.org

Parental control features for smartphones and devices:
Apple: Support.Apple.com/en-us/HT208982
Android: Families.Google.com/familylink

Body Image and Disordered Eating

"5 Ways to Stop Self-Criticism and Feel Better about Yourself Right
 Now," by Patricia Colli—A great article on body positivity
BeutifulMagazine.com/beutifulmagazine/2018/01/20/
 stop-self-criticism

*Getting Better, Bite by Bite: A Survival Kit for Sufferers of Bulimia
 Nervosa and Binge Eating Disorders*, by Urlike Schmidt, Janet
 Treasure, and June Alexander

The Healthy Teen Project—A compilation of organizations and
 professional references to help with eating disorders
HealthyTeenProject.com/resources

Healthy Relationships

Love Is Respect—The best resource I have found for identifying
 and supporting healthy relationships in the puberty years
LoveIsRespect.org

Tea and Consent—Great video for tweens and teens about consent
YouTube.com/watch?v=Exobo1GmYjs

Consent for Kids—A great video for younger children about consent
YouTube.com/watch?v=h3nhM9UlJjc

Rape, Abuse, and Incest International Network (RAINN)—The
 nation's largest anti-sexual violence organization
Rainn.org, 1-800-656-HOPE

LGBTQ+

Strong Family Alliance—A nonprofit organization focused on supporting parents of children in the LGBTQ+ community
StrongFamilyAlliance.org

PFLAG—An invaluable resource for parents and families of
LGBTQ+ children
PFLAG.org

*Parenting Your LGBTQ+ Teen: A Guide to Supporting, Empowering,
and Connecting with Your Child*, by Allan Sadac

*Gender Born, Gender Made: Raising Healthy Gender Non-Conforming
Children*, by Diane Ehrensaft, PhD

The Trevor Project—An excellent online resource for LGBTQ+ teens
TheTrevorProject.org

GLSEN—Resources for creating safer and more inclusive schools
GLSEN.org

National Center for Transgender Equality, Youth and Students—
Support and resources for transgender students
TransEquality.org/issues/youth-students

Books for Kids

*It's So Amazing! A Book about Eggs, Sperm, Birth, Babies, and Fami-
lies*, (for ages 7–10) by Robie Harris and Michael Emberley

*It's Perfectly Normal: Changing Bodies, Growing Up, Sex Gender, and
Sexual Health*, (for ages 10+) by Robie Harris and Michael
Emberley

A Celebration of Vulva Diversity, by Hilde Atalanta—Gift quality,
with playing cards and a special bag

REFERENCES

Abbey, Antonia, Tina Zawacki, Philip O. Buck, A. Monique Clinton, and Pam McAuslan. "Alcohol and Sexual Assault." *Alcohol Research & Health* 25, no. 1 (2001): 43–51. Pubs.NIAAA.NIH.gov/publications/arh25-1/43-51.htm.

Advocates for Youth. "Adolescent Sexual Health in Europe and the US—Why the Difference?" CDC.gov. Last modified May 15, 2015. NPIN.CDC.gov /publication/adolescent-sexual-health-europe-and-us-why-difference.

Ali, Syed Adel. "The Benefits of Journaling for Mental Health." Resources to Recover. April 24, 2021. rtor.org/2021/04/24/the-benefits-of-journaling -for-mental-health.

American Academy of Child and Adolescent Psychiatry. "Eating Disorders in Teens." Last modified March 2018. AACAP.org/AACAP/Families _and_Youth/Facts_for_Families/FFF-Guide/Teenagers-With-Eating -Disorders-002.aspx.

American Psychiatric Association. "Gender Affirming Therapy." Accessed November 2, 2021. Psychiatry.org/psychiatrists/cultural-competency /education/transgender-and-gender-nonconforming-patients/gender -affirming-therapy.

Arrien, Angeles. *The Four-Fold Way: Walking the Paths of the Warrior, Teacher, Healer, and Visionary*. San Francisco: HarperOne, 1993.

Atalanta, Hilde. A Celebration of Vulva Diversity. Self-published, 2019.

Boskey, Elizabeth, PhD. "The Anatomy of the Clitoris." Verywell Health. Last modified August 28, 2021. VerywellHealth.com/clitoris-anatomy -4774455.

Bowman, Christin P. "Women's Masturbation: Experiences of Sexual Empowerment in a Primarily Sex-Positive Sample." *Psychology of Women Quarterly* (December 2013). doi: 10.1177/0361684313514855.

Brenner, Grant Hilary. "Women's Sexual Pleasure, Orgasm, and Touching." *Psychology Today*. July 24, 2017. PsychologyToday.com/us/blog /experimentations/201707/womens-sexual-pleasure-orgasm-and -touching.

Brown, Cindy. "Vitamin B and Its Effect on Mental Health." CBT. April 25, 2020. CBTCognitiveBehavioralTherapy.com/vitamin-b-on-mental-health.

Carabotti, Marilia, Annunziata Scirocco, Maria Antonietta Maselli, and Carola Severi. "The Gut-Brain Axis: Interactions Between Enteric Microbiota, Central and Enteric Nervous Systems." *Annals of Gastroenterology* 28, no. 2 (April 2016): 203–9. NCBI.NLM.NIH.gov/pmc/articles/PMC4367209.

Castleman, Michael. "The Most Important Sexual Statistic." Psychology Today. March 16, 2009. PsychologyToday.com/us/blog/all-about-sex/200903 /the-most-important-sexual-statistic.

Centers for Disease Control and Prevention. "Anxiety and Depression in Children." Last revised March 22, 2021. CDC.gov/childrensmentalhealth /depression.html.

Centers for Disease Control and Prevention. "HPV Vaccine Recommendations." Last Reviewed March 17, 2020. Accessed November 2, 2021. CDC.gov/vaccines/vpd/hpv/hcp/recommendations.html.

Centers for Disease Control and Prevention. "Prevalence of Herpes Simplex Virus Type 1 and Type 2 in Persons Aged 14–49: United States, 2015–2016." National Center for Health Statistics. Last reviewed February 7, 2018. Accessed November 2, 2021. CDC.gov/nchs/products/databriefs /db304.htm.

Centers for Disease Control and Prevention. "Sexually Transmitted Infections Treatment Guidelines, 2021." Last reviewed July 22, 2021. Accessed November 2, 2021. CDC.gov/std/treatment-guidelines/default.htm.

Chaplin, Tara M. "Gender and Emotion Expression: A Developmental and Contextual Perspective." *Emotion Review* 7, no. 1 (January 2015): 14–21. doi: 10.1177/1754073914544408.

Chronobiology. "Sleep Deprivation in Teens Causes Anger, Depression and Lack of Energy." Accessed November 2, 2021. Chronobiology.com /sleep-deprivation-in-teens-causes-anger-depression-and-lack-of-energy.

Dawson, Connie, and Jean Illsley Clarke *Growing U.p Again: Parenting Ourselves, Parenting Our Children*. Center City, MN: Hazelden Publishing, 1998.

de Melker, Saskia. "The Case for Starting Sex Education in Kindergarten." PBS News Hour. May 27, 2015. PBS.org/newshour/health/spring-fever.

Donovan, Sophie. "'I Felt Suffocated': I Became Addicted to Porn at 10 Years Old and It Almost Ruined My Life." *The U.S. Sun.* September 26, 2020. The-Sun.com/lifestyle/1539930/i-became-addicted-to-porn-at-10.

Ehrensaft, Diane. *Gender Born, Gender Made: Raising Healthy Gender Non-Conforming Children.* New York: Experiment Publishing, 2011.

Feldman, Joshua. "Percentage of Films That Pass the Bechtel Test by Genre." Digital Image. Accessed November 2, 2021. i.redd.it/j4oqwl0ubz871.jpg.

Fjelstad, Margalis. "The Five Keys to Mindful Loving." Psychology Today. May 13, 2014. PsychologyToday.com/us/blog/stop-caretaking-the-borderline -or-narcissist/201405/the-five-keys-mindful-loving.

Flores, Andrew R., Jody L. Herman, Gary J. Gates, and Taylor N. T. Brown. "How Many Adults Identify as Transgender in the United States?" The Williams Institute at UCLA School of Law. June 2016. WilliamsInstitute .law.ucla.edu/publications/trans-adults-united-states.

Gallop, Cindy. "Make Love, Not Porn." Recorded December 2, 2009. TED video, 4:29. YouTube.com/watch?v=FV8n_E_6Tpc.

George, Tom. "It's Now Illegal in Norway to Not Label Retouched Photos on Social Media." June 30, 2021. Vice i-D (blog). i-D.vice.com/en_uk /article/88nmy4/norway-retouching-social-media-law.

Harris, Robie, and Michael Emberley. *It's Perfectly Normal: Changing Bodies, Growing Up, Sex Gender, and Sexual Health.* Somerville, MA: Candlewick Press, 2009.

Harris, Robie, and Michael Emberley. *It's So Amazing! A Book about Eggs, Sperm, Birth, Babies, and Families.* Somerville, MA: Candlewick Press, 2014.

Intersex Society of America. "How Common Is Intersex?" Archived 2008. ISNA.org/faq/frequency.

Jenco, Melissa. "Studies: LGBTQ Youths Have Higher Rates of Mental Health Issues, Abuse." *American Academy of Pediatrics News.* April 16, 2018. Publications.AAP.org/aapnews/news/13665.

John Hopkins All Children's Hospital. "What Is a Growth Spurt During Puberty?" John Hopkins Medicine. November 16, 2020. HopkinsAll Childrens.org/ACH-News/General-News/What-is-a-Growth-Spurt -During-Puberty.

Kastner, Laura S., and Jennifer Wyatt. *Getting to Calm: Cool-Headed Strategies for Parenting Tweens + Teens*. Seattle, WA: ParentMap Publishing, 2018.

Lembke, Anna. *Dopamine Nation: Finding Balance in the Age of Indulgence*. New York: Dutton, 2021.

Love Is Respect. "LGBTQ+ Relationships and Dating Violence." Accessed November 2, 2021. LoveIsRespect.org/resources/lgbtq-relationships -and-dating-violence.

Love Is Respect. "Relationship Spectrum." Accessed November 2, 2021. LoveIsRespect.org/everyone-deserves-a-healthy-relationship /relationship-spectrum.

Mahajan, Surbhi, MD. "8 Benefits of Honey on Skin: Know from Dermatologist." September 2, 2021. Accessed July 2021. Dermatocare .com/blogs/8-benefits-of-honey-on-skin-know-from-dermatologist.

Martinez, Gladys M. "Trends and Patterns in Menarche in the United States: 1995 through 2013–2017." Centers for Disease Control and Prevention. September 10, 2020. CDC.gov/nchs/data/nhsr/nhsr146-508.pdf.

Mastrangelo, Jamie. "When Does a Baby Develop Gender?" *Hello Motherhood*. June 13, 2017. HelloMotherhood.com/article/231357-when-does-a-baby -develop-gender.

Mayo Clinic Staff. "Growing Pains." Mayo Clinic. Accessed November 2, 2021. MayoClinic.org/diseases-conditions/growing-pains/symptoms-causes /syc-20354349.

Mayo Clinic Staff. "Gender Dysphoria." Mayo Clinic. Visited November 2, 2021. MayoClinic.org/diseases-conditions/gender-dysphoria/symptoms -causes/syc-20475255.

Mojtabai, Ramin, MD, PhD, and Mark Olfson, MD, MPH. "National Trends in Mental Health Care for US Adolescents." *JAMA Psychiatry* 77, no. 7 (March 2020): 703–14. doi: 10.1001/jamapsychiatry.2020.0279.

Moore, Kasey. "What Movie and TV Genres Perform Well in the Netflix Top 10s?" What's on Netflix. Published February 9, 2021. Whats-On-Netflix .com/news/what-movie-tv-genres-perform-well-in-the-netflix-top-10s.

National Institute of Health. "Teen Suicide: Understanding the Risk and Getting Help." September 2019. NIH News in Health. NewsInHealth.NIH .gov/2019/09/teen-suicide.

Niles, Andrea N., Kate E. Haltom, Catherine M. Mulvenna, Matthew D. Lieberman, and Annette L. Stanton. "Effects of Expressive Writing on Psychological and Physical Health: The Moderating Role of Emotional Expressivity." *Anxiety, Stress & Coping* 21, no. 1 (January 2014). doi: 10.1080/10615806.2013.802308.

Pagano, Robert. "The Relationship Between Hormones and Sleep." *Sleepline.* January 12, 2019. Sleepline.com/hormones.

Planned Parenthood. "Is Masturbation Healthy?" Visited November 2, 2021. PlannedParenthood.org/learn/sex-pleasure-and-sexual-dysfunction /masturbation/masturbation-healthy.

Planned Parenthood. "Puberty." Accessed June 2021. PlannedParenthood.org /learn/teens/puberty.

Planned Parenthood. "Transgender Identities." Accessed November 2, 2021. PlannedParenthood.org/learn/gender-identity/transgender.

Psychology Today Staff. "Porn Addiction." *Psychology Today.* Accessed November 2, 2021. PsychologyToday.com/us/basics/porn-addiction.

Racial Equity Institute. "The Groundwater Approach." RacialEquityInstitute .com/groundwaterapproach.

Sadac, Allan. *Parenting Your LGBTQ+ Teen: A Guide to Supporting, Empowering, and Connecting with Your Child.* Oakland, CA: Rockridge Press, 2021.

Savage, Adam. "Talking to My Kids about Sex in the Internet Age." Recorded October 28, 2013. The Moth MP3 audio, 10:59. TheMoth.org/stories /talking-to-my-kids-about-sex-in-the-internet-age.

Scheer, Roddy and Doug Moss. "Rises in Early Puberty May Have Environmental Roots." *Scientific American.* October 19, 2013. ScientificAmerican.com /article/rises-in-early-puberty-may-have-environmental-roots/.

Schmidt, Urlike, Janet Treasure, and June Alexander. *Getting Better, Bite by Bite: A Survival Kit for Sufferers of Bulimia Nervosa and Binge Eating Disorders.* Oxfordshire, UK: Routledge, 2015.

Schwarzbaum, Lisa. "The Bechtel Test: Can These Rules End Movie Sexism?" BBC. December 8, 2013. BBC.com/culture/article/20131207-can-three -rules-end-movie-sexism.

Scott, Jeffery. "A Closer Look at Carl Jung's Individuation Process: A Map for Psychic Wholeness." CEOsage. ScottJeffrey.com/individuation-process.

Short, Michelle A., Michael Gradisara, Leon C. Lacka, Helen R. Wright, and Hayley Dohnta. "The Sleep Patterns and Well-Being of Australian Adolescents." *Journal of Adolescence* 36, no. 1 (February 2013): 103–10. doi: 10.1016/j.adolescence.2012.09.008.

Singer, Katie. *Honoring Our Cycles: A Natural Family Planning Workbook.* White Plains, MD: Newtrends Publishing, 2006.

South Carolina Department of Mental Health. "Eating Disorder Statistics." Accessed November 2, 2021. State.sc.us/dmh/anorexia/statistics.htm.

Sutton, Jandra. "Everything You Need to Know about the G Spot." Healthline. June 5, 2018. www.healthline.com/health/g-spot-in-women#How-can -you-find-it?

Tello, Monique, MD, MPH. "Can Hormonal Birth Control Trigger Depression?" *Harvard Health Blog.* October 1, 2019. Health.Harvard.edu/blog/can -hormonal-birth-control-trigger-depression-201610172517.

Trans Hub. "What Is Gender Affirmation?" Accessed June 2021. TransHub .org.au/101/gender-affirmation.

Wells, Georgia, Jeff Horwitz, and Deepa Seetharaman. "Facebook Knows Instagram Is Toxic for Teen Girls, Company Documents Show." *Wall Street Journal.* September 14, 2021. WSJ.com/articles/facebook-knows -instagram-is-toxic-for-teen-girls-company-documents-show -11631620739?mod=article_inline.

World Health Organization. "Sexual Health." WHO.int/health-topics/sexual- health#tab=tab_1.

Worth, Tammy. "Does Vagina Size Matter?" WebMD. July 20, 2011. WebMD .com/women/features/vagina-size.

Youth.gov. "Adolescent Decision-Making Research." Accessed November 16, 2021. Youth.gov/youth-topics/adolescent-health/adolescent-decision -making.

Zambon, Veronica. "Can Transgender Women Have a Period?" Medical News Today. Last reviewed April 27, 2021. MedicalNewsToday.com/articles /can-trans-women-get-periods#summary.

Zane. Zachery. "Pornhub Just Dropped Some VERY Interesting Stats About Women's Porn Habits." *Men's Health.* December 11, 2019. MensHealth .com/sex-women/a30171574/pornhub-year-in-review-2019.

INDEX

Acknowledgments

This book was written on the ancestral homelands of the Lhaq'temish (Lummi) and Nuxwsa'7aq (Nooksack) Tribes.

I offer my heartfelt gratitude to every school leader who welcomed me into the classroom to guide students over the years. I especially thank Mike McCune of Cascades Montessori Middle School in Bellingham, Washington, for being the first to grant me this unique space as an independent sexuality educator.

I give my appreciation to the many supporters of Rooted Emerging, to all the families who joined our programs, to all the volunteers who made our offerings so magical, and to everyone who pulled me aside to ask for further support.

Grateful acknowledgment to the Sexual Health Advocates Group (SHAG), and especially Kara Eads for enduring support and alliance in so many ways.

To every client, young and old, who honored me with your trust, *thank you.*

About the Author

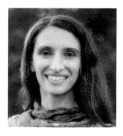

Vanessa Osage is a certified sexuality educator, consultant, speaker, and professional coach in love, sexuality, and human connections. In 2010, she founded Rooted Emerging, a nonprofit celebrating puberty rites of passage. In 2017, she was awarded the Kickass Single Mom Grant for her work in sexuality education and youth empowerment. She leads the social enterprise Love & Truth Rising and advocates for positive systemic change at The Amends Project. Her first book, *Can't Stop the Sunrise: Adventures in Healing, Confronting Corruption & the Journey to Institutional Reform*, available in print and audiobook, earned a 5-star review from IndieReader. Connect at VanessaOsage.com.

CPSIA information can be obtained
at www.ICGtesting.com
Printed in the USA
JSHW011246020322
23367JS00003B/5